Environmental Health and Occupational Safety

Pankaj Gupta

CRC Press
Taylor & Francis Group
Boca Raton London New York

CRC Press is an imprint of the
Taylor & Francis Group, an **informa** business

Designed cover image: Shutterstock

First edition published 2024
by CRC Press
2385 NW Executive Center Drive, Suite 320, Boca Raton FL 33431

and by CRC Press
4 Park Square, Milton Park, Abingdon, Oxon, OX14 4RN

CRC Press is an imprint of Taylor & Francis Group, LLC

ISBN: 978-1-032-73560-3 (hbk)
ISBN: 978-1-032-73562-7 (pbk)
ISBN: 978-1-003-46478-5 (ebk)

DOI: 10.1201/9781003464785

Typeset in Times
by MPS Limited, Dehradun

Environmental Health and Occupational Safety

The scope of occupational safety and health (OSH) has evolved gradually and consistently in response to variations that are socio-political or scientific, or generated by profit-seeking. In recent years, globalization of the world's economies and its impacts have been recognized as the greatest force for change in the domain of the workplace, and accordingly in the scope of OSH, both in positive and negative ways. OSH is a key element in achieving suitable working conditions and safety cultures.

Environmental Health and Occupational Safety is a quick, easy-to-consult comprehensive overview of the issues pertaining to environmental health and OSH. This book equips readers with occupational health risks and hazardous environments encountered in various industrial and workplace settings besides providing basic information on issues related to technology, management, regulatory compliance, and important topics like air, water, and vector-borne diseases.

Features:

- Clearly explains the key concepts of environmental health and OSH, and explores the benchmarks in the history of OSH.
- Talks about OSH as a sub-discipline of environmental health and its association with other disciplines.
- Comprehensive coverage of technical and scientific ideas underlying regulatory requirements and elucidates diverse facets of environmental health and OSH using flow charts and tabulations.
- The fact file at the beginning of each chapter highlights the key points on the themes covered in the chapter.

This book serves as a reference book for advanced students and researchers in the disciplines of environmental sciences, environmental health, eco-toxicology, pharmacology, public health, and OSH, as well as industry and government departments dealing with environmental regulations and directives.

Contents

Preface

Health and safety of an individual, family, community, and nation are intensely affected by occupational and environmental health issues. Environment professionals, environmentalists, and health and safety professionals play an important role in recognizing and preventing these issues. Thus, a deep understanding of the core concept of occupational and environmental health updates and endows these professionals to deliver their services more efficiently. Occupational safety and health (OSH) is the science of anticipation, recognition, evaluation, and control of hazards occurring in or from the workplace that can impair the health and well-being of workers, in view of the possible impact on the nearby communities and general environment. This domain is essentially enormous, covering a large number of disciplines and several workplace and environmental hazards. A variety of structures, skills, knowledge, and analytical capacities are desirable to coordinate and implement all *building units* that frame OSH systems so that the protection is extended to both workers and environment. The scope of OSH has evolved progressively and constantly in response to social, political, technological, and economic changes. In recent times, globalization and its repercussions have been perceived as the greatest force for transformation in the world of work, and consequently in the scope of OSH, both in positive and negative ways. Advancements in global trade, rapid technological development, momentous expansion in transport and communications, changing patterns of employment, changes in work practices, different occupation patterns, and size, structure, and life cycles of enterprises and new technologies produce new types and patterns of hazards, exposures, and risks. Demographic changes and population movements, and subsequent pressures on the global environment, affect safety and health in the world of work.

OSH deals with diverse facets of health and safety at workplace and has a strong focus on primary prevention of hazards. Its aim is to prevent accidents and harm to the workers from work-related activities. OSH is a key element in achieving sustained decent working conditions and strong preventive safety cultures, which include the basic principles of OSH, based on an approach of prevention and protection. The aim of OSH is to foster a safe and salubrious work-related environment. OSH protects even the general public who may be affected by the occupational environment. According to the World Health Organization, occupational health has a strong focus on primary prevention of hazards. The scope of OSH has evolved slowly and steadily in response to socio-political, scientific, and profitable deviations. In recent years, globalization of the world's economies and its impacts have been recognized as the greatest force for change in the domain of workplace, and consequently in the scope of OSH, in both positive and negative ways.

The book *Fundamentals of Environmental Health and Occupational Safety* is not only intended to support health and safety professionals and students in the health professions in recognizing and preventing occupational and environmental diseases and injuries in individuals and populations, but can turn out to be an essential reference for advanced students and researchers in the areas of environmental sciences, environmental health, occupational safety and health, etc., besides industry and government departments dealing with environmental regulations and directives. The book intends to make them understand the circumstances in which these diseases and injuries occur. It is an effort to underline the significance of safety and well-being of workers in occupational settings.

A single work cannot cover all topics in the vast field of environmental health and safety; hence, this book focuses on important themes indispensable for the promotion of OSH activities. It only offers an overview of occupational health risks and hazardous environments encountered in various industrial and workplace settings. The key workplace hazards include chemical agents such as dusts, heavy metals, and gases; physical agents like noise, radiation, and extremes of heat and cold; and biological agents. Guidelines and mitigation measures are suggested for managing each workplace hazard type.

– Pankaj Gupta

List of Abbreviations

Abbreviation	Full Form
ACGIH	American Conference of Governmental Industrial Hygienists
AD	Anno Domini
ADHD	Attention Deficit Hyperactivity Disorder
ADP	Adenosine Diphosphate
AIDS	Acquired Immunodeficiency Syndrome
AIHA	American Industrial Hygiene Association
Al	Aluminium
ARI	Acute Respiratory Infections
ARS	Acute Radiation Syndrome
As	Arsenic
Au	Gold
Ba	Barium
BCE	Before Christian Era
Be	Beryllium
Bi	Bismuth
BOD	Biochemical Oxygen Demand
CBT	Cognitive Behavioural Therapy
Cd	Cadmium
CHD	Coronary Heart Disease
CLL	Chronic Lymphocytic Leukaemia
CNS	Central Nervous System
CO	Carbon Monoxide
Co	Cobalt
CO_2	Carbon Dioxide
COD	Chemical Oxygen Demand
COPD	Chronic Obstructive Lung Diseases
Cr	Chromium
CTDs	Cumulative Trauma Disorders
Cu	Copper
CV	Cardiovascular
CVD	Cardiovascular Disease
DALYs	Disability-Adjusted Life Year
DDT	Dichloro-Diphenyl-Trichloroethane
DDT	Dichlorodiphenyltrichloroethane
DNA	Deoxyribonucleic Acid
DO	Dissolved Oxygen
eg	For Example
EC	Electrical Conductivity
ECG	Electrocardiography
EMFs	Electromagnetic Forces
FAO	Food and Agriculture Organization

Fe	Iron
GAD	General Anxiety Disorder
GDP	Gross Domestic Product
GHGs	Greenhouse Gases
GI	Gastrointestinal
GMOs	Genetically Modified Organisms
HABs	Harmful Algal Blooms
HC	Hydrocarbons
HCN	Hydrocyanic Acid
HCS	Hazard Communication Standard
Hg	Mercury
HIV	Human Immunodeficiency Virus
HMs	Heavy Metals
ie	That is
ILO	International Labour Organization
IQ	Intelligence Quotient
IR	Ionizing Radiation
LCM	Lymphocytic Choriomeningitis
Li	Lithium
Mg	Magnesium
MI	Myocardial Infarction
MM	Multiple Myeloma
Mn	Manganese
MRI	Magnetic Resonance Imaging
MRSA	Methicillin-Resistant Staphylococcus Aureus
MS	Mass Spectrometry
MSDs	Musculoskeletal Disorders
NCDs	Non-Contagious or Non-Communicable Diseases
NHL	Non-Hodgkin Lymphoma
Ni	Nickel
NMR	Nuclear Magnetic Resonance
NO	Nitric Oxide
NOx	Nitrogen Oxides
OA	Osteoarthritis
OEL	Occupational Exposure Limit
OHS	Occupational Health and Safety
OPIDN	Organophosphate-Induced Delayed Neuropathy
OSHA	Occupational Safety and Health Agency
PAHs	Polycyclic Aromatic Hydrocarbons
PAs	Pyrrolizidine Alkaloids
Pb	Lead
PCBs	Polychlorinated Biphenyls
PCs	Phytochelatins Compartmentation
PEB	Pro-Environmental Behaviour
PM	Particulate Matter
PNS	Peripheral Nervous System

PPE	Personal Protective Equipment
ppm	Parts per million
Pt	Platinum
PTSD	Post-Traumatic Stress Disorder
PVC	Polyvinyl Chloride
QMRA	Quantitative Microbiological Risk Assessment
RADS	Reactive Airways Dysfunction Syndrome
RBCs	Red Blood Cells
RDS	Respiratory Distress Syndrome
RNA	Ribonucleic Acid
RSIs	Repetitive Strain Injuries
RT	Radiation Therapy
SARS	Severe Acute Respiratory Syndrome
Sb	Antinomy
SDGs	Sustainable Development Goals
SDI	Species Diversity Index
Sn	Tin
SO_2	Sulphur Dioxide
SPM	Suspended Particulate Matter
Sr	Strontium
TB	Tuberculosis
TDS	Total Dissolved Solids
Te	Tellurium
Ti	Titanium
TIX	Tetrodotoxin
Tl	Thallium
U	Uranium
UK	United Kingdom
UN	United Nations
UNEP	United Nations Environment Programme
UNICEF	United Nations Children's Fund
USA	United States of America
UV	Ultra Violet
VOC	Volatile Organic Compounds
VSM	Vascular Smooth Muscle
WBCs	White Blood Cells
WHO	World Health Organization
Zn	Zinc
alpha	Alpha
beta	Beta
gamma	Gamma

Author Biography

Holding a Doctorate in Life Sciences from Himachal Pradesh University and a Faculty Member in the Department of Environment Sciences, HP University, Dr. Pankaj Gupta is presently a Fellow at the Indian Institute of Advanced Study, Shimla. He is an empanelled consultant of NABARD and HPPCL for conducting Environmental and Social Impact Assessment and baseline studies. He is a member of various academic and professional bodies, viz. Life Member, Society for Environment and Development; Member, Ethno-botanical Society, Lucknow; and Member, International Society for Ethno-pharmacology. He is also an Editor of Confluence of Knowledge, an international refereed journal, since 2013 and Indian Correspondent, Journal of Folk Art of Eurasia. He is a content writer of IGNOU's learning material of M.Sc. (Environmental Sciences) and has contributed ten units. Dr. Gupta is the Chief Editor of the SAGES CHRONICLES, a monthly e-magazine of SAGES. He was awarded the Best Young Researcher Award for the year 2022 by Himachal Pradesh University on its Foundation Day.

He was awarded Certificate of Appreciation by the Vice-Chancellor, HPU for drafting the *Heerak Jayanti Drishtipatr*: Diamond Jubilee Vision Document, 2030 and Chief, Institute of Complex Researches in Great Altai, Altai State Technical University, Barnaul City, Russian Federation for his outstanding research and academic work.

Dr. Gupta has completed more than 15 research projects and 12 consultancies. He has authored and edited 23 books (with national and international publishers), and published 50 research papers in journals of repute and 24 chapters in edited volumes.

1 Environmental Health

"You cannot achieve environmental security and human development without addressing the basic issues of health and nutrition"

—Gro Harlem Brundtland

FACT FILE

According to the UNEP *Healthy Environment, Healthy People* report:

- lack of access to clean water and sanitation causes 58 percent of cases of diarrheal diseases in low and middle-income countries
- unsafe water, inadequate sanitation, or insufficient hygiene result in 3.5 million deaths worldwide, representing 25 percent of premature deaths of children younger than 14
- mental health issues rank among the ten largest non-fatal threats in most nations

According to the World Health Organization (WHO):

- environmental stressors are accountable for 12–18 percent of all deaths in the 53 countries of the WHO Europe region
- effects of air pollution on humans are significant, viz. air pollution causes 29 percent of all global deaths from lung disease; 24 percent of all global deaths from stroke; 17 percent of all global deaths and disease from acute lower respiratory infection
- environmental issues account for more than 12.6 million deaths each year
- global environmental issues account for more than 12.6 million deaths each year
- more than 100 illnesses and injuries can be directly linked to environmental health concerns
  - Air pollution is the world's largest single environmental risk to health and nearly 7 million people across the world die each year because of daily exposure to poor air quality
  - Air pollution is the single largest environmental health risk and is linked with heart disease, stroke, lung disease, and lung cancer.
  - Children under 15 years are mainly affected, with 36 percent of all deaths accounted for environmental factors

DOI: 10.1201/9781003464785-1

- About one-third of the world's population lacks access to proper sanitation services
- Every day, more than 2,200 children die because of diseases caused by poor water quality
- Even in developed countries, environmental factors play a major role in burden of disease
- Exposure to air pollution is estimated to result in premature deaths
- Exposure to excessive noise causes annoyance, sleep disturbance, and related increase in the risk of hypertension and cardiovascular disease
- Health surveys across the world state that more than 780 million people don't have access to clean drinking water
- The financial costs of environmental-related health risks are generally in the range of 5–10 percent of GDP, with air pollution taking the highest toll
- 784 million people across the world still drink dirty water
- With exposure to pesticides, the rate of brain cancer has increased by up to 20 percent

1.1 INTRODUCTION

Maintaining a healthy environment is vital for helping people live longer and enhancing their quality of life. By improving environmental health, communities can decrease exposure to disease, in addition to pollutants that have a toxic effect on the body. According to the new UNEP report entitled '*Healthy Environment, Healthy People*', the degradation of the environment – the air we breathe, the food we eat, the water we drink, and the ecosystems which nurture man – is estimated to be accountable for at least a quarter of the global total burden of disease. The *2030 Agenda for Sustainable Development* and its *Sustainable Development Goals* (SDGs) reflect that a healthy environment is integral to the realization of basic human rights, including the right to life, health, food, water, sanitation, and quality of life.

A clean environment is important for the health and well-being of all living organisms. Man has co-evolved with nature and has remained dependent on it for sustenance; yet, with the development and anthropogenic activities, human health has been adversely affected by changing environments including climate change, heat waves, floods, and vector-borne diseases. At a broader level, climate change, biodiversity loss, and land degradation have not only threatened ecosystem services, such as access to freshwater and food production, but the health of all living beings. Human health and well-being are closely linked to the state of the environment. The natural environment provides fundamental needs in terms of clean air and water, fertile land for producing food, besides energy and material inputs for production. At the same time, the environment acts as an important pathway for human exposure to polluted air, noise, and hazardous chemicals. Exposure to hazardous chemicals is one of the main concerns, for the human population is exposed to a variety of chemicals in their routine lives, via polluted air and water, consumer products, and diet. Some of the hazardous chemicals persist in the environment and bio-accumulate in the food chain. This increases concerns about the health impacts of exposure to chemicals over one's lifetime, mainly during vulnerable life stages, such as early childhood, pregnancy, and old age. Therefore, improving the quality of the environment can prevent disease and improve human health. Environmental health isn't just an issue of an individual's wellness; it's a matter of community welfare. A number of environmental problems can impede human health and wellness. These issues include:

1. **Air Pollution:** Impact of air pollution on humans is an important public health concern, for exposure to air pollution increases both morbidity and mortality. Air pollutants include gases, solid or liquid particles that remain suspended in the air and have detrimental or toxic effects. Some of the most unsafe air pollutants include car and truck exhaust, and emissions from industrial processes. But, many natural air pollutants, for instance, pollen and mould spores act as natural air pollutants that pose threats to human health by causing asthma and allergies.
2. **Chemical Pollution:** Human beings are exposed to diverse chemicals in one way or the other, which in turn affect their health. More precisely, we seek to protect human and environmental health from exposure to potential toxins. According to the World Health Organization (WHO), more than 1.6 million deaths in 2016 were because of exposure to chemicals. Moreover, heavy metals and toxins find their way into the water supply and later into the food chain.
3. **Climate Change and Natural Disasters:** Another environmental issue with life-threatening consequences for human health is climate change, together with the increasing incidence of natural disasters. According to the National Environmental Health Association, climate change is the biggest human health threat of the 21st century that disrupts the natural world in a number of ways that can affect health and increase vulnerability to disease. Increasing temperature, erratic rains, and runoff often result in greater susceptibility to nervous and respiratory diseases. Moreover, climate change increases the frequency of natural disasters, viz. wildfires, hurricanes, cyclones, and droughts often having an intimidating effect on families and communities and sometimes results in loss of life.
4. **Diseases Caused by Microbes:** Health implications due to microbes, viz. bacteria, viruses, and fungi are another area of public health concern. Trillions of microbes occur both in the environment and the human body. Though most of them have no negative health effects, many of them perform important biological functions. Harmful microbes, commonly known as pathogens or germs, can infect human beings and animals thus causing illness. Eating is one of the main means wherein human beings come in contact with microbes. *E. coli*, a type of bacteria found in the environment and foods, can cause respiratory illness, urinary tract

infections, and other adverse health effects. Numerous harmful microbes in the soil can also cause diseases and humans can come in contact with them by ingesting or inhaling them. Tetanus and botulism are examples of diseases caused by soil-borne microbes.

5. **Global Environmental Issues:** Soil pollution, UV radiation, and biodiversity loss are the global issues that have the greatest impact on communities, mainly the underprivileged and those already having vulnerabilities.
6. **Inaccessibility to Proper Healthcare:** Another environmental factor that contributes to disease and poor health outcomes is lack of access to proper healthcare services. Economic insecurity, defective conveyance to medical facilities, and lack of awareness and education contribute to inaccessibility to healthcare.
7. **Infrastructure Problems:** Infrastructure problems can have a major impact on community health; for example, poorly maintained roads increase the risk of car accidents; lack of access to clean drinking water poses threats of waterborne diseases; lack of local healthcare infrastructure capable of giving vaccinations, poses threats of exposure to numerous communicable and non-communicable diseases, having implications on human health.
8. **Poor Water Quality:** The health implications due to polluted water are glaring. A number of factors contribute to water contamination, including industrial waste and pollution, inaccessibility to proper water treatment, poor hygiene services, and outdated sanitary fixtures. There has been growing evidence suggesting that exposure to natural environments can be linked with mental health. It has been established that clean air and water, hygiene and vegetation, and a safe workplace can enhance quality of life and reduce mortality and morbidity. A healthy environment promotes healthier lifestyles, improves the productivity of workers and their families, improves the life of women, children, and aged, and is vital to mental health. The determinants of health and well-being in hierarchical order (in ascending order) include:
   - People (age, sex, and genetic factors)
   - Lifestyle (diet, physical activity, and balance between workplace-life)
   - Community (social capital, networking)
   - Local economy
   - Activities (working, playing, running)
   - Built Environment
   - Natural Environment
   - Global Ecosystem (climate change, biodiversity, etc.)

1.1.1 Right to a Healthy Environment

On October 8, 2021, the UN Human Rights Council adopted a resolution identifying the right to a clean, healthy, and sustainable environment as an important human right. While this right is already known in more than 150 nations, its international recognition paves the way for its successful incorporation into international law for its stronger implementation. The right to a healthy environment has gradually developed since the 1970s when it was first mentioned during the Stockholm Declaration of 1972. Its first Principle states:

> "Man has the fundamental right to freedom, equality and adequate conditions of life, in an environment of a quality that permits a life of dignity and well-being".

The Stockholm Declaration acted as a facilitator for identifying the right to a healthy environment at the national and regional levels. According to the UN:

> Currently the right to a healthy environment "is included in regional human rights treaties and environmental treaties binding more than 120 States. It enjoys constitutional protection in more than 100 States and is incorporated into the environmental legislation of more than 100 States. In total, 155 States have already established legal recognition of the right to a healthy and sustainable environment."

At the national level, Portugal was the first nation to treasure this right in its constitution in 1976. Since then, the right to a healthy environment has promptly spread to other constitutions. The international recognition of the right to a healthy environment is less progressive, as until now many nations have shown reluctance in adopting a legal binding for recognizing such a right. Thus, the right to a healthy environment remained devoid of legal force in international environmental law. Apart from the aforementioned Stockholm Declaration, the Rio Declaration (1992) affirmed that:

> Human beings are at the center of concerns for sustainable development. They are entitled to a healthy and productive life in harmony with nature.

1.2 HEALTHY ENVIRONMENT: BASIC REQUIREMENTS

The term '*healthy environment*' is a huge one, having diverse meanings. Sometimes, it is believed that the environment that is healthy for one population may not be amiable for the other. Thus, to create a healthy environment, it is important to consider human beings, and other living organisms, viz. animals, microbes, insects, and plants. The healthy environment thus refers to the human environment that would pose few health hazards. According to most dictionaries, environment is the sum total of adjoining living conditions, which means all physical things, all growing things, all structures, objects, and chemicals.

The issues of a healthy environment have deeper implications and it is believed that people often forget the structures where they live and houses, buildings, and roads are taken for granted for these cannot simply be ignored in creating a healthy environment. Studies have shown that buildings and structures can have an impact on the environment; for instance, schools located near busy roads are subjected to higher levels of pollution that affect human health. Not only the urban environment, but the rural environment is also subjected to various ecological problems; for instance, the excessive use of pesticides and chemical fertilizers has greater risk of causing respiratory diseases and cancer. Reviewing the environmental problems helps people understand which problems are of great concern. The answer to how to create a healthy environment is not possible to find from a single source, instead it comes to humans in scraps, like a mystery. Each human has a responsibility of deciding how to fit those bits together to create a better world. Environmental health, a branch of environmental sciences and a sub-branch of public health focuses on the relationship between man and environment. It promotes human health and is an essential component of public health. Certain factors, such as clean air, water, food, accommodation, and climate need to be considered to attain health and prosperity. Ensuring a healthy environment to live in is one of the basic necessities.

1.2.1 Environmental Factors and Causes Affecting Health

The indicators of a healthy environment and well-being are:

Safe Drinking Water: It is the basic necessity of life. Contaminated water is one of the biggest health concerns of human beings.

Environmental Toxicity: A number of chemicals, gases, toxins, and persistent organic pollutants exist all the time in the environment, which poses threats not only to the health of human beings, animals, and plants but also natural resources such as soil and water. These health impacts manifest in a range of disorders varying from skin infections to genetic disorders. Additionally, a number of pesticides enter the food chain and affect the living organisms.

Air Pollution: Air pollution, both outdoor and indoor, is one of the most serious environmental problems that affect all living beings. Industrial activities and vehicular traffic have resulted in emission of large amounts of noxious gaseous and particulate matter, which is affecting the respiration system of living organisms.

Urbanization: It is concerned with the expansion of urban areas and wherever poorly developed, urbanization has resulted in increased release of urban waste and uncontrolled consumption of water.

Climate Change: Climate change is the topmost threat to the human race, which not only causes environmental and economic damage, but increases the incidence of natural disasters, such as flooding, earthquakes, and avalanches.

Sufficient and Safe Food: Safe and peaceful settlements, housing and community infrastructure govern human health. It has been seen that civil violence disrupts housing and well-being. Therefore, a peaceful atmosphere is one of the key factors responsible for a healthy environment.

Stable Global Environment: Human health and ecosystem are closely linked. However, global environmental factors also contribute to the well-being of the community; for example, long-range transport of air pollutants, trans-boundary movement of water pollutants, and climate change have implications on larger populations and even across borders and continents. The man-nature link is inseparable. Clean water, air, and healthy food are the basic necessities for human survival. Human civilization has a close connection with the environment. A healthy environment connotes a healthy life, for it reduces the risk of diseases. Proper food, shelter, clean air, and water improve the quality of life and increase life expectancy. Any change in the environment will have direct consequences on sustenance; for example, if the temperature increases then the food security decreases, which consecutively will cause malnutrition and disease.

1.2.2 Determinants of Health

There are three basic determinants of health:

- the social and economic environment
- the physical environment, and
- the person's individual characteristics and behaviours

Income and social status govern health, for higher income and social status are linked with better health. The greater the gap between the richest and poorest people, the greater will be the variances in health. Likewise, educational status too plays a significant role in governing health status, because low education level is associated with poor health, more stress, and less self-confidence.

Physical environment, including safe drinking water, unpolluted air, healthy place of work, safe dwellings, communities, and roads all contribute to good health. Employment and working conditions also determine health, for employed people are healthier, particularly those who have more control over their working conditions. Social support networks also play a significant role in healthy living; for example, greater support from families, friends, and communities contribute to better health. Culture, customs, traditions, and the beliefs of a family or a community also affect health. Moreover, genetics has a role in governing life expectancy, well-being, and the chance of developing diseases. Personal behaviour and coping skills, including a balanced diet, keeping oneself active, avoiding smoking and alcohol consumption, and proper dealing with life's stresses and challenges all affect health. The availability of good healthcare services, access, and use of services that prevent and treat disease also influences health. Besides this, gender also determines the health status of an individual, for men and women suffer from different types of diseases at different ages.

1.3 ENVIRONMENTAL QUALITY

Environmental Quality is a term that refers to the varied characteristics like air and water pollution, noise, access to open space, and visual effects of buildings, and the potential effects which such characteristics may have on physical and mental health (caused by human activities). Environmental Quality:

- is a set of characteristics of the environment, either universal or local, as they impact human beings and other organisms;
- is a measure of environmental condition relative to the condition of one or more species;
- includes the natural and built environment, such as noise, air and water quality, and the potential effects which such features may have on physical and mental health

Thus, environmental quality refers to the quality of the total environment, and not just the natural environment, because it is a measure of the health of the environment itself and of the outcomes it has on the health, comfort, and mental state of the human beings that inhabit it. The natural environment consists of the air, water, and land that constitute the planet, plants, and animals, while the built environment is the environment created by human beings for themselves. The quality of the environment thus depends on the fact of how the natural environment affects human health and comfort. It is also dependent on the natural resources on which human beings sustain. It is essential to maintain and protect environmental quality to:

- attract visitors and new residents
- be respectable curators of the planet
- conserve community resources
- create a better quality of life
- fascinate new, eco-friendly corporate initiatives that withstand economic health
- increase the aesthetic character of a community
- maintain ecosystems
- protect endangered species
- safeguard community from ecological disasters
- stop people from taking actions they'll regret later
- sustain a community's history
- uphold the health of a community and its members

The quality of the environment has to be maintained when:

- it's specifically threatened
- there's a community development initiative
- there's a new commercial, industrial, or housing development
- there's an environmental crisis
- there's media attention to the environment
- resources are accessible

The following can play an important role in ensuring environmental quality:

- Anyone who is cognizant of the consequences of environmental quality
- Businesses and corporations
- Community/environmental activists
- Local, national, and international environmental organizations
- Local, state, and federal officials
- Those directly affected by the environmental quality (this category can include people with very different approaches to the environment, viz. those whose living depends on it; those whose business is environmental quality or the study of the environment; people who use the natural environment for recreation and spiritual support; architects and environmentally conscious developers)

1.4 HUMAN EXPOSURE TO NOXIOUS SUBSTANCES IN THE ENVIRONMENT

Numerous facets of the environment affect human health for environmental hazards increase the risk of disease, including cancer, heart disease, and asthma. Table 1.1 shows how different aspects of environment can affect human health.

Table 1.2 highlights some of the major environmental disease/outbreaks in the last century.

TABLE 1.1
Environmental Exposures and Related Human Health Implications

Environmental Exposure	Health Implications
Asbestos	• Respiratory problems • Lung cancer • Mesothelioma
Climate change	• Communicable diseases (giardiasis and salmonellosis; heat stroke) • Injury/death from extreme heat/cold, sores, floods, and fires • Intensification of respiratory diseases • Population dislocation • Vector-borne diseases • Water pollution due to increased sea level
Crowded habitation/poor ventilation/smoke	• Acute/chronic respiratory disease • Lung cancer
Exposure to naturally occurring toxic substances	• Poisoning
Exposure to UV radiation	• Eye cataracts • Little exposure results in Vitamin D deficiency, causing rickets, osteoporosis and osteomalacia

(Continued)

TABLE 1.1 ***(Continued)***

Environmental Exposures and Related Human Health Implications

Environmental Exposure	Health Implications
	• Melanoma • Non-melanoma skin cancer
Exposures to vehicular/industrial air pollution	• Cancer • Loss of IQ in children • Respiratory diseases
Hazardous substances	• Burns • Dermatitis • Poisoning
Household congestions	• Communicable diseases, including lower respiratory infections
Improper water resource management/poor drainage	• Vector-borne diseases
Lead	• Developmental delays and behavioural problems in children • Increased blood pressure in adults
Natural resources degradation/natural hazards	• Injury and death
Noise	• Cardiovascular problems • Hearing loss • Insomnia • Psychophysiological problems
Outdoor air pollution	• Cardiovascular disease • Lung cancer • Respiratory disorders
Ozone depletion	• Cataracts • Compromised food production • Skin cancer
Polluted water	• Gastrointestinal problems • Eye, ear, nose, and throat infections
Population migration/encroachment	• Infectious diseases (for example, HIV/AIDS, Ebola) • Vector-borne diseases
Second-hand smoke exposure	• Low birth weight, sudden unexpected death in infancy in infants • Asthma, lower respiratory infections, middle ear infections in children • Cardiovascular problems, stroke, lung cancer in adults
Unfit drinking water sanitation and solid waste disposal, improper hygiene (hand washing)	• Gastrointestinal problems • Vector-related diseases (for example, malaria, schistosomiasis, and dengue)
Vectors including mosquitoes, ticks, etc.	• Malaria, dengue fever, Rickettsial disease

TABLE 1.2
Major Environmental Disease Outbreaks

Country	Year	Environmental Hazard	Disease	Causalities
South-east Turkey	1955–1961	Hexachlorobenzene in seed grains	Porphyria; neurological disease	3,000
USA cities	1960–1970	Lead in paint	Anaemia, behavioural and mental effects	Many thousand
Toyama, Japan	1950s	Cadmium in rice	Kidney and bone disease (Itai-itai disease)	200 with severe disease, many more with slight effects
London, UK	1952	Air pollution with sulphur dioxide and Suspended Particulate Matter (SPM)	Increase in heart and lung disease manifestations	3,000 deaths, many others ill
Minamata, Japan	1956	Methylmercury in fish	Neurological disease (Minimata disease)	200 with severe disease, 2,000 suspected
Fukuoka, Japan	1968	Polychlorinated biphenyls (PCBs) in food oil	Skin disease, general weakness	Several thousand
Iraq	1972	Methylmercury in seed grains	Neurological disease	500 deaths, 6,500 hospitalized
Madrid, Spain	1981	Aniline or other toxin in food oil	Various symptoms	340 deaths, 20,000 cases
Bhopal, India	1985	Methyl isocyanate	Acute lung disease	2,000 deaths, 200,000 poisoned
California, USA	1985	Carbamate pesticide in watermelons	Gastrointestinal, skeletal, muscle, autonomic and central nervous system effects (Carbamate illness)	1,376 reported cases of illness resulting from consumption, 17 severely ill
Chernobyl, USSR	1986	Iodine-134, Caesium-134 and -137 from a reactor explosion	Radiation illness (including increases in cancer and thyroid diseases in children)	300 injured, 28 died within 3 months, more than 600 cases of thyroid cancer
Goiánia, Brazil	1987	Caesium-137 from an abandoned cancer therapy machine	Radiation illness (follow-up of *in utero* exposures continuing)	Some 240 people were contaminated and 2 died
Peru	1991	Cholera epidemic	Cholera	139 deaths, many thousand ill

1.5 NATURE OF ENVIRONMENTAL HEALTH HAZARDS

Environmental health hazard refers to a problem or issue, wherein environment has implication on the safety and well-being of living organisms. Present day environmental health issues are the consequences of climate change, deforestation, and pollution, which are the resultant of anthropogenic activities. These activities produce hazardous substances which remain in the air, soil, and water and consequently affect the health of the environment. Generally, the environmental contaminants are classified as:

- **Carcinogen** (cancer-producing agents, for instance, formaldehyde, asbestos, radon, vinyl chloride, and tobacco)
- **Endocrine Disruptor** (chemicals interfering with the body's endocrine system and producing adverse developmental, reproductive, neurological, and immune effects in both human beings and animals; for example, pharmaceuticals, dioxin and dioxin-like compounds, arsenic, Polychlorinated Biphenyls (PCBs), DDT and other pesticides, and plasticizers such as bisphenol A).
- **Mutagen** (material inducing genetic changes (mutations) in the DNA, for instance, radioactive substances, such as radon and nitrous acid)
- **Neurotoxin** (substance causing an adverse effect on the chemistry, structure, or function of the nervous system, for example, lead and mercury)
- **Teratogen** (substance causing physical defects in a developing embryo, for example, alcohol and cigarette smoke)

1.5.1 Classification of Environmental Health Hazards

On the basis of the causative factor, the environmental health hazards are classified as (Figure 1.1):

1. **Physical hazards** (including processes occurring in the natural environment and can potentially harm human health; for example, radiation, body stress, limited spaces, electricity, heat, heights, noise, natural disasters, and vibration can have health implications). Health risks are posed due to

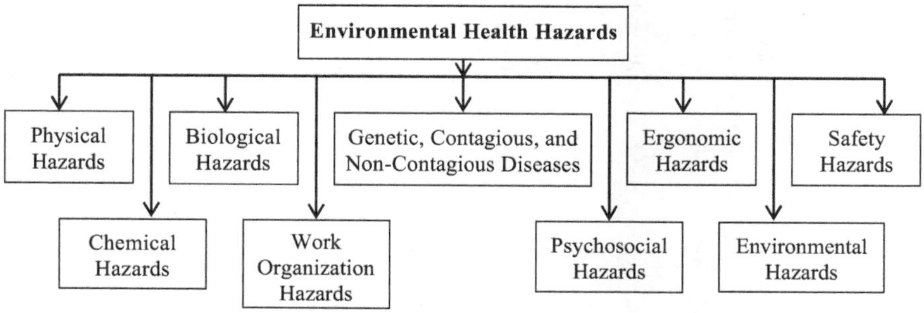

FIGURE 1.1 Classification of environmental health hazards.

physical agents or natural substances at workplace. When a person works in an environment in extreme temperatures, viz. too hot or cold or high levels of humidity, thermal radiation, or simply in the sun, a physical hazard may occur threatening health and safety. Some physical hazards, such as explosions or radiation, can arise from natural or human sources. Every day, human beings are exposed to natural radiation sources, for example, the UV radiation of the sun. Human beings are also exposed to radiation from man-made sources like medical X-rays and smoke detectors. Exposure to low levels of radiation from watching television or construction materials is also common. All these physical hazards have health implications. Extreme working conditions at workplace can all harm workers, causing breathing problems, audible loss, and malignancy, among other problems. Workers who are exposed outside in the sun for a prolonged period of time can suffer physical hazards which can cause long-term effects to their health. Physical hazards can be any factors within the environment that can harm the body without necessarily touching it. Of all hazards, physical hazards are least evident. Physical hazards include:

- Electric shocks
- Exposure to sunlight/UV rays
- Extremes temperature, viz. hot and cold
- Gases under pressure
- Loud noise
- Radiations, including ionizing and non-ionizing

Another common physical hazard can be a natural disaster, for example, a cyclone or earthquake, for it puts the well-being and safety of man at risk. It may arise naturally as earthquakes, wildfires, landslides, etc., or extreme weather. These may also arise due to human structures or activities (accident, building collapse, injury due to mechanical equipment, body strain due to repeated movements, etc.).

2. **Chemical Hazards** refer to a non-biological substance having the potential to harm or cause a negative impact on human health and life. Chemical hazards occur when a worker is exposed to any chemical preparation in the workplace in any form (solid, liquid, or gas). These hazards are caused by toxic, corrosive, inflammable, and explosive chemical agents and pose health risks to workers. Human beings are exposed to a variety of chemicals at home, workplace, or even in the air which can have both short and long-term health effects when absorbed by the body. Chemical hazards may be the result of using flammable or combustible, explosive, oxidizing, shock-sensitive, substances. These may be carcinogens, irritants, sensitizers, teratogens, or toxins. Air pollutants (such as second hand smoke or carbon monoxide), heavy metals, and pesticides are other hazard-producing substances. Human beings are exposed to these contaminants from a variety of residential, commercial, and industrial sources. The four major routes of entry include:

- Absorption (through the eyes or skin)
- Inhalation (through the respiratory system)

- Ingestion (through the gastrointestinal tract via the mouth)
- Injection (through the skin or cut/wound)

Chemical hazards can be present in the following:

- Liquids like cleaning products, paints, acids, and solvents – mainly if hazardous chemicals are in un-marked vessels/ampules
- Vapours/fumes due to welding or exposure to solvents
- Gases like acetylene, propane, CO, helium, H_2S gas
- Hazardous products and flammable materials like gasoline, solvents, and explosive chemicals
- Pesticides

3. **Biological hazards** can be defined as harmful or dangerous impacts arising from the interface of organisms within the natural environment. The biological hazards, generally known as biohazards, can be due to biological substances that could cause harm to humans. Biological hazards are caused after exposure to harm or disease while working with animals, people, or infectious plant materials. It may include bacterial infections, viruses, diseases, or other forms of pathogens, with a lethal impact on human beings. Cholera, influenza, malaria, tuberculosis, etc., are examples of biological hazards. These hazards are infectious diseases caused by pathogens (disease-causing organisms or infectious particles) such as bacteria, fungi, parasitic worms, protozoa, viruses, prions, animal/insect bites, fungi/moulds, animal and bird droppings plants, microbes, sewage, blood, and body fluids. These are more common in schools, day-care facilities, colleges and universities, hospitals, laboratories, nursing homes, etc. These hazards can cause diseases and allergic reactions. While talking about biomechanical hazards, it is important to identify that biomechanics is related to more than manual handling. Biomechanics use laws of physics and engineering concepts to define movements and forces acting on the body parts during routine activities and may cause a Musculoskeletal Disorder (MSD) resulting in damage to muscles, bones, connective tissues, nerves, or blood vessels. Physical factors governing the risk of injury from biomechanical hazards include exertion, movement and repetition, body posture, exposure, and vibration.
4. **Psychosocial hazards** are associated with the psychological and social conditions of the workplace rather than the physical conditions. Employees are likely to be exposed to a mixture of occupational psychosocial hazards and risk factors, including stress, fatigue, bullying, violence, aggression, harassment, and burnout, which can be detrimental to the health of workers and compromise their security. Psychosocial hazards can create stress, which can cause psychological or physical harm. Stress itself is not an injury; but if employees are frequently stressed, over a long time, or the level of stress is high, it can cause harm, which may manifest as anxiety, depression, post-traumatic stress disorder, sleep disorders; while physical harm may include musculoskeletal injuries, chronic disease or fatigue-related injuries. Psychosocial hazards may interact or combine to create new, changed, or higher risks.

5. **Genetic, Contagious, and Non-Contagious Diseases:** A genetic disease is caused by a deviation in the genome of a person, which may range from minor to major, ranging from a discrete mutation in a single base of DNA to a gross chromosome abnormality including the addition or subtraction of an entire chromosome or set of chromosomes. While some diseases, such as cancer, may also be placed in the category of genetic disorders, they can also be caused by environmental factors. Recessive gene disorders manifest in some environments, where environmental factors play an important role. At times, a disease is a result of a combination of genetic and environmental factors. Many cancers and some other diseases are the result of environmental triggers. Sickle cell disease is a collective term for a group of blood diseases caused by inheritance of haemoglobin S. The pathological process in sickle cell disease is caused by the sickling phenomenon. In the deoxy state haemoglobin S molecules aggregate into long polymers which are aligned to form liquid crystals called tactoids.

   In the presence of tactoids, the normal disc-shaped, easily deformable red cell is transformed into the characteristic sickle-shaped cell that gives this condition its name. The sickling phenomenon harms the membrane of RBC and it gradually becomes rigid. Such cells are seized in the reticulo endothelial system and rapidly demolished, causing haemolytic anaemia. A second major disturbance in sickle cell disease arises because of altered flow properties of sickled red cells. There is an increase in blood viscosity linked with small vessel stasis and obstruction, which eventually leads to vasocclusive crises and eventually to permanent organ damage. Moreover, patients suffering from sickle cell disease have a tendency to bacterial infection because of a combination of other factors. Besides the impact of direct environmental factors, the occurrence of non-communicable adult disease is determined by non-genetic and genetic developmental factors; for example, attention deficit hyperactivity disorder (ADHD), a developmental disorder that is mainly characterized by "the co-existence of attentional problems and hyperactivity. In this case, neurotrophic factors participate in the neurogenesis, survival, and functional maintenance of brain systems, and are an implication of genetic predisposition to ADHD. During the past few decades, experimental evidence has suggested that environmental factors influence cellular proliferation attrition in an organ-specific manner. Mostly, the transmission rates are considerably lower than expected. In such cases, and in disorders with no genetic background, environmental factors seem to influence and/or cause disease onset, progression, and outcome. Thus, environmental factors are threats to health, and monitoring them is linked with the community's environmental health. They include:

   - **Air quality:** pollen and pollution leading to respiratory diseases or cancers
   - **Ecological conditions:** favouring disease vectors (endemic and exotic vectors)

- **Environmental disruptions:** floods, droughts, storms, fires, earthquakes, volcanoes
- **Invasive biota:** (viruses, bacteria, etc.), their hosts and vectors
- **Monitoring and management of municipal, agricultural, and industrial outflows** in the environment (gases, liquids, solid wastes)
- **Water quality:** biotic and abiotic contaminants; integrity of water transport and treatment infrastructure

Research has shown that environmental factors are accountable for approximately 24 percent of the global burden of disease and 23 percent of all deaths. About 25 percent of the deaths in developing nations and 17 percent of deaths in developed countries are due to environmental factors and children are the worst victims of the same. Nearly 24 percent of the deaths in children under 15 are due to diarrhoeal diseases, malaria, and breathing problems, all of which are caused due to environmental factors. The global burden of disease is the result of:

- Climate change
- Exposure to indoor smoke and toxic elements
- Outdoor air pollution
- Sanitation and poor hygiene
- Unsafe water and poor hygiene

While advancement has been made with regard to availability of drinking water, the situation in many Asian countries remains bad as far as sanitation is concerned. Currently, almost 2.5 billion people lack public health facilities, the poorest being in South Asia. According to UNICEF, 67 percent of people in rural India still practice open defecation. Among some South-East Asian countries, the proportion of population lacking access to water and sanitation is still very poor. The linkage with disease is evident as unsafe water and sanitation add to 94 percent of the diarrhoeal diseases. Drinking water and sanitation have not received proper attention even though the benefits of the two can go beyond the health and economic development of a nation. Setting the top priority for allocating resources and including water, sanitation, and hygiene must be the prerequisite of nation-building. Moreover, indoor and outdoor pollution also affects human health. Each year, an estimated 42 percent of respiratory tract infections are linked with indoor and outdoor pollution including second-hand smoke. Long-term exposure to Suspended Particulate Matter (SPM) from indoor burning of solid fuel is a major cause of respiratory diseases like Chronic Obstructive Lung Disease (COPD) especially among children. According to WHO, outdoor air pollution contributes to 800,000 deaths each year globally and about 60 percent of them are from Asia, due to consumption of fuel, motor vehicles, industries and burning of waste. These issues are causing ischaemic heart disease, acute respiratory infections, asthma, and lung cancer. There is evidence which reveals that change in environment due to development has negative health implications; for example, construction of the Aswan Dam in Egypt increased the incidence of malaria and schistosomiasis. Likewise, deforestation has resulted in soil erosion and flooding.

Nearly 42 percent of malaria in Asia and Africa is due to environmental factors, such as land use, deforestation, and water resource management. Similarly, cultivation of rice, rearing of pigs, breeding vectors, and exposure to unsafe water play an important role in transmission of acute encephalitis syndrome. Environmental factors considerably add to the pandemic like dengue and transmission of schistosomiasis. Cancer, believed to be the second leading cause of death around the world, has more incidence in developing countries and accounts for more than two-thirds of deaths. Of the annual cases of cancer each year, 19 percent are due to the environment. Smoking is responsible for 71 percent of deaths because of lung cancer. Stomach cancer, the second most common cancer due to *H. pylori* infection, is linked with poor sanitation and overcrowding conditions. Recent studies in Indian states have revealed a high incidence of cancer in Punjab, the reason being increased use of pesticides, the traces of which are even found in soil and water. Exposure to indoor smoke due to burning of fossil fuels or tobacco smoke or smog can initiate an asthma attack, mainly during the winter. As far as the prevalence of COPD is concerned, more than one-third of deaths due to COPD are due to environmental causes.

The on-going environmental factors such as climate change have substantial impacts on health and well-being of mankind. Non-Contagious or Non-Communicable Diseases (NCDs), also known as chronic diseases, are believed to be caused due to a combination of genetic, physiological, environmental, and behavioural factors. Cardiovascular diseases (such as heart attacks and stroke), cancers, chronic respiratory diseases, and diabetes are the main NCDs, which extremely affect people in underdeveloped and developing nations, where more than three-quarters of global deaths occur due to NCD. NCDs affect people of all age groups, regions, and nations. Children, adults, and the elderly are equally vulnerable to the risk factors associated with NCDs and are driven by forces that include rapid unplanned urbanization, globalization of unhealthy lifestyles and ageing. Unhealthy diet and lacking physical activity lead to increased BP, increased blood glucose level, raised blood lipid level, and obesity.

6. **Environmentally-related Hazards:** This category includes a number of diseases, which are caused by the organisms present in the environment. Trachoma, or the preventable blindness caused by the bacterium *Chlamydia trachomatis*, spreads easily by contact with an infected person's hands or clothing, or by flies coming in contact with the eyes or nose of an infected person. Infected individuals do not immediately go blind; instead, the disease manifests slowly. Blindness from trachoma strikes adults in their prime years, obstructing their capability to care for themselves and their families.

   Onchocerciasis, also known as river blindness, infects approximately 18 million people, of which the majority live in sub-Saharan Africa. Worldwide, over 120 million people are at risk of contracting river blindness. Communities living near the fast-moving streams of Africa are at high risk since these act as breeding grounds for the Simulium black fly.

Infected flies carry larvae of the filarial parasitic worm *Onchocerca volvulus* from person to person. Larvae enter the skin after the bite of black fly, move throughout the body, and then die, resulting in a variety of health problems including skin rashes and de-pigmentation, itching, and skin nodules. Visual impairment and blindness occur if larvae enter the eye.

Guinea worm disease, known as *Dracunculiasis,* is caused by the parasitic worm *Dracunculus medinensis*. It is transferred after ingestion of stagnant water contaminated with the larvae of guinea worm. The larvae after entering the body, migrate into body tissues, and develop into adult worms. Female worms move through tissue, causing intense pain, and finally emerge through the skin, producing oedema, a blister and ultimately an ulcer, accompanied by fever.

Schistosomiasis is acquired after contact with parasitic worms released by freshwater snails. Inside the body, the larvae develop into worms. Female worms release thousands of eggs which are passed out of the body and discharged into freshwater by urination or defecation. They migrate to snails and restart the life cycle. Eggs entrapped in the body migrate to specific organs and inflict major damage, for instance, scarring, and tearing of bladder and kidneys.

Hookworm, roundworm, and whipworm result in soil-transmitted intestinal infections and are among the most common infections in the world. These infections are linked with poverty and poor sanitation. Ascariasis, an intestinal infection caused by *Ascaris lumbricoidesart* is most prevalent in warm tropical and sub-tropical climates in Sub-Saharan Africa and Southeast Asia. The disease flourishes in areas with poor sanitation and poorly irrigated crops treated with wastewater. It is the most common human worm infection. Whipworms, caused by *Trichuris trichiura,* cause weakness, anaemia, rectal prolapse, and even delay growth in children. Improved sanitation and hygiene are critical to the elimination of these diseases.

Hookworms, caused by the soil transmitted parasitic worms *Necator americanus and Ancylostoma duodenale* affect approximately 576–740 million individuals worldwide. Infected individuals typically experience gastrointestinal symptoms. Lymphatic filariasis, also known as elephantiasis, is common in tropical and sub-tropical climates, both in rural and urban areas where infected mosquitoes breed. Lymphatic filariasis is transmitted when infected mosquitoes bite humans and pass microfilariae into the skin. Larvae migrate through the body and settle in the lymphatic system, where they lay eggs which pass into the blood, where the worms can live for up to six years. Once these die, they cause severe disfiguring ailments, including the swelling or hardening of the skin, severe lymphedema of extremities or genitals.

Environmental hazards are caused due to frequently changing erratic and extreme weather and climate conditions. These hazards are mostly out of control. These include extreme temperatures (heat and cold), extreme precipitation (rain and snow), harmful levels of noise and radiation, pollution (air and chemical), unstable infrastructure, biological hazards, violence, and dangerous animals. Thus, environmental health not only focuses on avoiding illness and injury at workplace, but it also strives to promote worker health and well-being. Administrations and governments can encourage healthy practices and behaviours for their employees by providing fitness centres, a restroom, or a canteen serving nutritious food and encouraging healthy social interface and eating habits for keeping them physically active. In this chapter an effort has been made to discuss the cause and effect of some workplace hazards.

7. **Ergonomic Hazards:** These safety hazards occur when a specific type of work, body position, and working condition puts a strain on your body. They are the toughest to recognize because these are not noticed immediately after the strain on the body or harm that these hazards pose. Short-term exposure may cause "sore muscles" the subsequent day or in the days following the strain, but long-term exposure can result in severe long-term impacts. Ergonomic hazards include difficult movements, mainly if these are recurring, extreme vibration, frequent lifting, improper sitting/standing/working posture, improperly adjusted workstations, and chairs and using too much force, mainly frequently.
8. **Safety Hazards:** Safety hazards affect employees who work directly with machinery or on construction sites. Unsafe working conditions can cause injury, illness, and death. These include:
   - Anything that can cause falls
   - Contact with carelessly moving machinery parts
   - Electrical hazards due to improper wiring
   - Restricted spaces
   - Something that can cause falls, for example, working from heights, including ladders, scaffolds, roofs, or any high work area.
9. **Work Organization Hazards:** Safety hazards or stressors can cause short-term effects like stress or long-term effects like strain. These hazards are related with workplace concerns, for example, workload, lack of control, and/or respect; the examples of these hazards include workload demands, workplace violence, social support or relations, and sexual harassment.

1.6 WORKPLACE PSYCHOLOGY AND ENVIRONMENT

The workplace environment is used to define the elements that include the physical and social milieu in which an employee works. It is an all-inclusive concept including the physical setting, occupational attributes, organizational features, and extra-organizational traits, such as work-home relationships. When assessing the psychological impact of the working environment, the impact on an individual's cognizance and behaviours must be considered. While exploring the impact of the workplace environment, two factors must be considered:

- Firstly, this impact is influenced by the interpretation a worker makes regarding their surroundings.

- Secondly, it may be a result of the grouping of a number of circumstances, rather than one factor.

Numerous areas contribute to the staff satisfaction and welfare in healthcare. These include individual factors, such as burnout, personality and family/work conflicts, and job-related factors, such as amount of work, shift type, duration, and stress level.

1.6.1 Pro-Environmental Behaviour

Pro-environmental behaviour (PEB), also known as green-, sustainable-, or eco-friendly behaviour, is defined as a behaviour in which individuals take self-protective actions toward the environment. It includes sensibly engaging with outdoors or recycling household waste together with adaptive response to the impact of climate change, water or energy conservation, or shifting modes of travel to buying an electric vehicle. With anthropogenic climate change the term "*climate change adaptive behaviour*" has come into being, which is defined as any behaviour individuals can engage in to buffer the hazardous impacts of climate change that leads to the benefits of climate-change-induced mitigation and sustainability. PEBs, as part of climate change adaptive behaviour contribute to environmental sustainability.

1.6.2 Environmental Health Management

Environmental health as a branch of public health deals with how the living, working, and leisure environment can affect human health. Emergencies and disasters can occur at anyplace in the world, affecting human health, life of people, and infrastructure supporting them. Health risks in emergencies can arise from an effect of disaster on the physical, biological, and social environment, including water contamination, sanitation, and waste-management systems. Emergencies may also increase the risk of chemical and radiation exposures. WHO recommends preventing environmental health risks through:

- precautionary measures, such as community awareness, early warning systems, construction of disaster-prone health facilities, and resilient water and sanitation systems;
- preparedness, including firming of policies for disaster management and evolving disaster response plans;
- disaster response, including supervision of hazardous materials and recovering infrastructure loss; and
- retrieval processes, such as renovating resilient water and sanitation infrastructure.

As part of the International Health Regulations, WHO identifies, confirms, and issues warnings for incidents of public health concern, including those involving environmental health hazards. It has been researched and shown that crowded conditions enable transmission of diseases including tuberculosis, influenza, meningitis, acute respiratory infections (ARI), diarrheal diseases, and measles. Children living in congested houses are mostly more vulnerable to ARI. Crowding can also cause psychological distress in children and encourage physical violence. It is recommended that each child must have a minimum of 1 m^3 of space in the home. Damp housing conditions may shelter viral and bacterial agents, along with house dust mite, which can cause respiratory problems. Damp conditions also encourage the growth of mould and are thought to be a contributory factor to rheumatism and arthritis. Indoor air pollution can be mainly hazardous to health because it is released in close proximity to people. The "rule of 1000" states that a pollutant released indoors is 1000 times more likely to reach people's lungs than a pollutant released outdoors. Indoor air pollution due to open fires, unsafe fuels, and ineffective stoves for cooking and/or heating probably denotes the single most serious health impact from air pollution. The burning of domestic biomass fuels, coal, and kerosene by underprivileged communities both in developing and developed countries, can lead to extremely high levels of indoor air pollution. This poses risks to the respiratory health of women and young children.

In addition to fumes from combustion, indoor pollutants from building materials, paints, solvents used in the home and environmental tobacco smoke affect human health. Indoor air quality is also affected by outdoor pollution sources, e.g. garages, petrol stations, manufacturing plants, burning charcoal, and quarrying. Sources of biological contamination of food are diverse and include polluted water, dirty hands, flies, pests, domestic animals, besides dirty cooking pots and utensils, and human and animal excretion. *Bacillus cereus*, *Staphyloccocus aureus,* and *Clostridium perfringens* are food-borne pathogens that cause diseases often accompanied by diarrhoea and gastroenteritis/stomach pains. Infection due to *Clostridium botulinum* is rare but draws public attention owing to its high case-fatality rate. Many chemical hazards in food are produced naturally by organisms in the environment, such as *Aspergillus flavus*, which produces aflatoxin. Others are inherent components of food itself, as in the case of poisonous mushrooms. Pollutants such as lead, cadmium, and polychlorinated biphenyls (PCBs) in air, water, and soil also produce high levels of toxic chemicals in food with serious health implications if ingested chronically. Likewise, mycotoxins, plant toxins and marine bio-toxins can contaminate food and are hazardous to health.

1.6.3 Environment and Value Education

Value education is expected to bring about a sustainable way of life. Education, both through formal and non-formal processes, must address understanding of:

- Causes of ecological degradation
- Environmental, natural, and cultural values
- Equitable use of resources
- Human heritage
- Management of Common Property Resources
- Social justice

Values are a set of principles or standards of behaviour that are regarded as desirable, important, and held in high esteem by society.

Environmental Values: Every human being has feelings for different facets of his or her environment. The ecological values go beyond valuing a river for its water, a forest for its wood and non-timber forest products, or the ocean for its fish. Environmental values are intrinsic in feelings that bring about compassion for conserving nature. This is a more spiritual, and traditional value. There are several writings and sayings across different religions of the world that support the concept of the oneness of entire creation, respecting and valuing different elements of nature. Throwing away large quantities of non-degradable waste is damaging the environment and the value system can play a significant role in preventing this. Pro-environmental actions must start from the domain of individuals and go up to a community. Environmental values must stress on the significance of conserving ancient structures. The distinctive architecture, sculpture, artworks, and crafts of ancient civilizations are invaluable environmental assets, which enlighten each one of us for:

Valuing nature and respecting diverse human cultures, because it is the responsibility of each one of us to protect life in its glorious forms. There is not only a need to protect natural ecosystems but also to protect the rights of people.

Valuing culture for every culture is linked closely with nature and no one has the right to disturb and disrupt life. Everyone must appreciate that diverse cultures across the world have a system of traditional knowledge of their own environments which is based on a deep sense of respect for nature.

Human heritage, for the planet Earth itself is a heritage and its preservation is a growing environmental concern. The ancient civilizations and their valuable contribution in the form of architectural assets, created in an eco-friendly manner teach the principles of conservation and glorious heritage.

Equitable use of resources for it is based on socially and environmentally consciousness of individuals. There is a need to change consumption patterns and switch over to sustainable lifestyles. Indigenous societies around the world have been judiciously using resources with an idea of conserving the same for the future generations as well. The same idea must percolate and prevail in the future as well. Their concept of managing commonly-owned resources has been the key principle responsible for environmental conservation and the same may continue to play a significant role in the future as well.

Ecological degradation for valuable ecological assets can turn into serious environmental problems, if not managed properly. The transformation from traditional land-use patterns to more intensive utilization has resulted in environmental degradation. These values must form a part of a new conservation ethic.

Social justice to respect and value the diverse aspects of nature and society, because if the poor are not respected, they will rebel and it will spread terrorism.

Therefore, the developing world will face an environmental crisis, unless the people value and protect nature.

BIBLIOGRAPHY

Barton, H. and Grant, M. (2006) A health map for the local human habitat. The Journal of the Royal Society for the Promotion of Health 126(6):252–261.
Bayley, J. (1991) Health and safety at work. British Dental Journal 170(10):364–365.
Carman, J. P. and Zint, M. T. (2020) Defining and classifying personal and household climate change adaptation behaviors. Global Environmental Change 61:102062.
Cutler, R. (1991) Health and safety at work. British Dental Journal 170(7):251.
Hernberg, S. (1992) Introduction to Occupational Epidemiology. Philadelphia: Lewis Publishers.
Hui-Yi, Y., Kou-Huang, C. and Kow-Tong, C. (2018) Environmental determinants of infectious disease transmission: A focus on one health concept. International Journal of Environmental Research and Public Health 15(6):1183.
Krajhanzl, J. (2010) Environmental and pro-environmental behavior. School and Health, Health Education: International Experiences 21:251–274.
Levy, B. S. and Wegman, D. H. (1994) Occupational Health: Recognizing and Preventing Work-Related Disease. Boston: Little Brown.
Nichols, T. (1998) Health and safety at work. Work, Employment & Society 12(2):367–374.
Prüss-Üstün, A. and Corvalán, C. (2006) Preventing Disease through Healthy Environments. Towards an estimate of the environmental burden of disease. Geneva: World Health Organization.
Rosenstock, L. and Cullen, M. R. (1994) Textbook of Clinical Occupational and Environmental Medicine. Philadelphia: Saunders.
Schneider, F., Lesko, W. and Garrett, W. (1980) Helping behavior in hot, comfortable cold temperatures. Environment and Behavior 12(2):231–240.
Scott, R. M. (2020) Chemical Hazards in the Workplace (e-book). Boca Raton: CRC Press.
Spurlock, B. (2017) Physical Hazards of the Workplace. Boca Raton: CRC Press.
Steg, L. and Vlek, C. (2009) Encouraging pro-environmental behavior: An integrative review and research agenda. Journal of Environmental Psychology 29:309–317.
Van Valkengoed, A. M. and Steg, L. (2019) Meta-analyses of factors motivating climate change adaptation behavior. Nature Climate Change 9:158–163.
Wilson, H. G. E. and Agius, R. M. (1994) Health and safety at work. BMJ 309(6948):198–199.
Zalesny, M. D. and Farace, R. V. (1988) Job function, sex and environment as correlates of work perceptions and attitudes. Journals of Applied Social Psychology 18(9):179–202.

2 Occupational Safety and Health

"An incident is just the tip of the iceberg, a sign of a much larger problem below the surface"

Anonymous

FACT FILE

- Nearly 3.5 billion people or nearly half of the world's population are workers
- Each year, approximately 160 million new cases of occupation-related diseases occur worldwide
- People above 60 years of age suffer the greatest number of fatal falls
- More than 125 million people around the world are exposed to asbestos in the workplace
- Approximately 160 million non-fatal work-related diseases and nearly 317 million non-fatal occupational accidents occur per year, which means that every 15 seconds a worker dies from a work-related accident or disease, and every 15 seconds, 151 workers have a work-related accident
- Approximately 4–6 percent of GDP and annual economic losses occur from illnesses and injuries due to unhealthy and hazardous working conditions
- Women, children, and migrant workers are least protected and most affected due to occupational health hazards
- More than two million people die every year from work-related diseases and injuries
- Only 5–10 percent of workers in developing nations and 20–50 percent of workers in industrial nations have access to adequate occupational healthcare services
- Annually, work-related injuries and diseases result in the death of approximately two million people globally, which is larger than the annual deaths from malaria
- Some occupational risks, for instance, injuries, noise, carcinogenic agents, airborne particles, and ergonomic risks are accountable for a considerable portion of burden of chronic diseases with 37 percent of cases of back pain, 16 percent of cases of hearing loss, 13 percent of cases of chronic obstructive pulmonary disease, 11 percent of cases of asthma, 8 percent of

DOI: 10.1201/9781003464785-2

cases of injuries, 9 percent of cases of lung cancer, 2 percent of cases of leukaemia, and 8 percent of cases of depression
- Annually, 12.2 million people, mostly in the developing nations, die from non-communicable diseases while still in the active working age
- Among the occupational injuries, falls are the second leading cause of accidental injury deaths across the globe
- Every year more than 680,000 individuals worldwide die from falls of which over 80 percent are in low- and middle-income nations
- All forms of asbestos are carcinogenic to human beings
- Deaths and injuries take a mainly heavy toll in developing nations, where a large segment of the population is involved in hazardous activities, such as farming, construction, fishing, and mining

2.1 INTRODUCTION

Occupational safety and health is among the most vital aspects of human interest. It deals with the acclimatization of workplace settings by the workers for the advancement and maintenance of the highest degree of physical, mental, and social well-being of workers. With rapid industrialization and agricultural development in developing nations, occupational health and safety (OHS) is becoming a global concern. Many nations are switching over from manual labour to service mechanization in the industrial sectors, for instance, manufacturing, mining, and farming; as a result, probable occupational health consequences are expected. The ravenous aspirations of man for technical innovation have opened the doorways for refined technology and equipment not only in the industrial sector but also in the service and commerce sector. This has perpetually been linked with a change in the entire composition of the workforce as well as a rise in the engagement of women. Hence, the associated health issues linked with occupation are likely to change, for instance, more emphasis on job-related psychosocial factors is more desirable in the service sector, which will be a new challenge for OHS practice in most of the developing and underdeveloped nations for the cutting-edge means to handle such problems and the expertise are still not available in these countries. Occupational health in developing nations is seen both at a local and national level. Locally, the positive impact of occupational health services may be seen in decreasing morbidity and work-related injuries. Furthermore, this also means fewer fatalities for employers and workers because there will be a reduced cost of reimbursement. The lack of skilled labour, mainly so in nations where there is a shortage of skilled labour, is of great importance.

Developing a safe, healthy, and salubrious working environment in the interest of workers, employers, government, and the public at large is becoming critically imperative. Though it seems easy and undemanding, this idea has not yet gained significant worldwide appreciation. Hundreds of millions of people around the globe are working in an environment that produces ill-health and/or is insecure and hazardous. Every year, work-related injuries and diseases kill nearly two million people worldwide, which is larger than the global yearly deaths from malaria. Each year, nearly 160 million new cases of occupation-related diseases occur worldwide, including respiratory and cardiovascular diseases, cancer, hearing loss, and musculoskeletal, reproductive, mental, and neurological disorders. In recent years, increasing numbers of workers are complaining about psychological stress due to overload, resulting in sleeplessness, despair, tiredness, and burn-out syndromes, with growing risks of cardiovascular diseases. Even in progressive economies, a large proportion of workplaces are not examined frequently for OHS.

2.1.1 Historical Background

The concept of OHS evolved with the beginning of civilization. Efforts have been made by the kings and monarchs for the safety of their workers; for instance, Hammurabi, king of Babylon in the 18th century BC, issued laws to ensure the safety of his workers. Likewise, ancient Egyptians laid down laws about the number of working hours for workers involved in building the pyramids. There is a broad description of diseases prevalent in working areas, for instance, health issues arising due to the inhalation of flying dust while sharpening weapons made from granite in granite quarries. From the very beginning, man has been making consistent efforts to understand and comprehend problems arising in the working place. The origin of OHS concerns can also be linked with the industrial revolution that took place in the late 18th century to early 19th century, and resulted in the emergence of cotton mills, semi-automated factories, and iron industries. Although the industrial revolution resulted in economic development, it had a negative impact on the health and safety of the workers. Men and women workers were exposed to harmful gases, toxins, acids, extreme heat and cold temperatures, and light and sound that had a detrimental impact on their physical, social, and mental well-being. This drew the interest of scholars, thinkers, and social workers to address the issues of industrial health and hygiene. Consequently, acts, legislations, and policies were formulated across the globe, with the objective of ensuring good health and safe work environments for all workers. Each nation has its own act and policy on OHS. Work-related disease issues have been identified for a long time. Some of the milestones achieved in this regard are presented in chronological sequence:

- Hippocrates in 400 BC for the first time observed that workers who handled mercury sulphide suffered from illness in ancient Greece. He described the symptoms of lead poisoning among miners and metallurgists.
- Pliny the Elder (23–70 AD) was a Roman legislator who wrote about the workers who used to fasten animal bladders on their mouth for guarding themselves from dust. He also detected hazards of asbestos and cinnabar, the ore of mercury.
- Ulrich Ellenborg (1473), a German physician, recognized the dangers of metal fumes and described the signs and precautionary methods.
- Paracelsus (1493–1541), a Swiss physician wrote a treatise on occupational diseases and described the lung diseases among miners and recognized the cause of vapours released from metals. He is best known today as the '*Father of Toxicology*' for his observations of dose and response:

"All substances are poisons; there is none which is not a poison. The right dose differentiates a poison and a remedy"

- In the 1540s, Barracelios, in Austria, gave a description of pulmonary disease among mining workers.
- In Bohemia in 1556, Georgius Agricola wrote about the diseases among mining workers and the role of a well-ventilated working environment and protective equipment for preventing the incidence of respiratory diseases caused after exposure to gases and dust. He was a physician who appointed in the mining town of Jochimstral in the Swiss mountains. He wrote *De Re Metallica*, a comprehensive discourse addressing every aspect of mining, smelting, and refining. He suggested the need to keep aeration for miners, and described '*asthma*' among workers who worked in sooty and smoky mines.
- Bernardino Ramazzini (1633–1714), an Italian physician, known as the "patron saint of industrial medicine", conducted a study on industrial diseases and wrote a book *De Morbis Artificium Diatriba* (*The Diseases of Workmen*) that described the symptoms of mercury and lead poisoning and other occupational diseases. He also wrote about the pathology of silicosis and suggested safeguards to avoid hazards. He advised physicians to learn about occupational diseases by analysing the work environment, and insisted them to always ask their patients "Of what trade are you?"
- Sir George Baker (1722–1809) discovered that '*Devonshire colic*' was caused by lead contamination in cider.
- Percival Pott (1714–1788), a London physician, was the first to link occupational exposure to cancer, mainly scrotal cancer among chimney sweeps, caused by soot. Later, he also established that scrotal cancer is caused after exposure to Polycyclic Armoatic Hydrocarbons present in coal soot.
- Sir Humphrey Davy (1788–1829) investigated problems of mine explosions and developed the first miner's safety lamp.
- In 1858, John Stanhaos presented the first mask to prevent exposure to gases and vapours.
- In 1802, labour and safety laws were issued in the United Kingdom
- In 1833, an entity was formed to inspect factories and ensure the prevention of occupational accidents of child labourers
- In 1840, the Royal Commission published a report on the status of workers in the mining industry, which revealed the high percentage of terrible accidents in an industrial setup, as well as the hazardous and non-secure working environment.
- In 1844, came the Law of Mines which forced mine owners to improve the working environment
- In 1889, limits were laid down concerning exposure to moisture and CO_2 in cotton factories in the UK
- In 1883, Bismarck launched the first social insurance legislation in Germany and the Workers' Compensation Act 1884

- In 1910, Allen Hamilton was designated as the first scientist in industrial toxins, and a pioneer in the field of toxicology and occupational health
- Dr. Alice Hamilton (1869–1970) was the first woman faculty member at Harvard University (1919) and a social activist who worked to improve OHS. Her autobiography '*Exploring the Dangerous Trades*' details her experiences in the mines and mills across America.
- An industrial renaissance occurred between 1920 and 1930 and was accompanied by the development and growth of industrial health in public health, which led to the formation of the American Conference of Governmental Industrial Hygienists (ACGIH) in 1938 and the American Industrial Hygiene Association (AIHA) in 1939.
- In 1953, the British Occupational Health Society (BOHS) was founded
- In 1970, Occupational Safety and Health Agency (OSHA) was established under the Ministry of Labour to ensure the safety and health of workers, by setting and executing standards and providing training, awareness-generation, education, and assistance.
- In 1972, the OSHA Training Institute was started to train individuals on safety and health in the public and private sectors.

2.1.1.1 Tragedies that Stirred a Change

Workplace disasters of the early 1900s led to brutality and consequently a regulation to protect workers. *The Triangle Shirtwaist Fire* was probably the most important event leading to the regulation of occupational safety. The Triangle Shirtwaist Company was a New York City "sweatshop" where dozens of mostly young female immigrant workers were busy to cut and sew shirtwaists. Shirtwaists were popular ladies garments of the time, particularly for working women. Sweatshop workers are paid low wages as they work overly long hours in unsanitary and unsafe conditions. In 1911, The Triangle Shirtwaist Company factory caught fire, and 146 workers died in the upper floors of this "fireproof" building. Fire exits were inadequate or locked to keep the workers at their workstations, and they were unable to flee; many victims jumped from the windows to their deaths. Later, the disaster led to 36 laws ameliorating the state labour codes.

The *Gauley Bridge Disaster of 1930*, also known as the *Hawks Nest tragedy*, was America's worst industrial disaster. Construction of the Hawks Nest tunnel near Gauley Bridge, West Virginia, triggered huge exposures to silica dust. At least 476 men died and 1,500 incapacitated by silicosis. Silica exposures were so high men died from acute silicosis from only two months of exposure. Pneumatic boring equipment and rock high in silica content increased the risk. Economic factors of the Great Depression forced the men to work in insalubrious environments. Occupational safety and health is a cross-disciplinary area and it interacts with other disciplines. Its relationship with other branches of science and medicine is depicted in Figure 2.1.

On average, the people of an economically active society spend about one-third of their time at the workplace. The status of employment and working environment plays a significant role in governing the health of a society. A healthy working environment not only offers social protection and personal development prospects

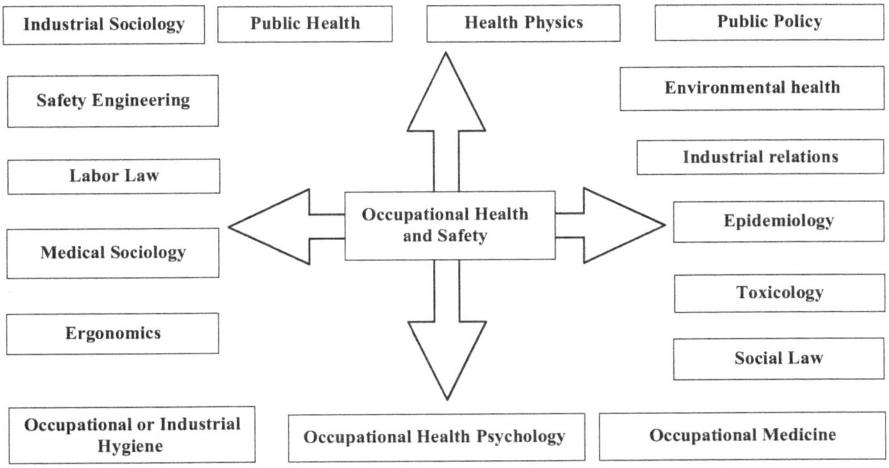

FIGURE 2.1 Relationship of OSH with other branches of science.

but security from physical and psychosocial hazards. A healthy working environment improves the social relations and self-esteem of employees and brings about positive health impacts. The health of the workers is an indispensable pre-condition which in turn affects household income, output, and economic development. Hence, restoring and sustaining working capacity is imperative for health services. Health risks at the workplace, for example, heat, noise, dust, hazardous chemicals, unsafe machines, and psychological stress, bring about occupational diseases and magnify other health complications. Employment conditions and the status at the workplace also affect health. People working under stress or in risky employment environments are likely to smoke more, exercise less, and have an unhealthy diet. Besides general healthcare, all workers – and mainly those in high-risk occupations, need healthcare services to evaluate and decrease exposure to occupational risks, and medical investigation for initial detection of occupational diseases and injuries. The most common occupational diseases are chronic respiratory diseases, musculoskeletal disorders, noise-induced hearing loss, and skin problems.

2.1.2 Factors Governing Worker's Health

Occupation-related non-communicable diseases (NCDs) in addition to cardiovascular diseases and depression caused by occupational stress, have a cumulative impact on the incidence of long-term illness and absenteeism from work. Occupational NCDs include occupational cancer, chronic bronchitis, and asthma caused due to air pollution in the workplace and radiation. Despite these diseases, in the majority of countries, physicians and nurses are not trained effectively to address occupational health problems and many nations do not offer postgraduate education in occupational health. Prevention strategies in this regard emphasize education, training, creating secure and protected environments, and executing effective policies for risk reduction.

2.1.3 Defining Occupational Health

Occupational health is a sub-discipline of public health meant to promote and maintain the highest degree of physical, mental, and social well-being of labour in all professions. Its purpose is to:

- maintain and promote the health and working capacity of workers;
- improve the working environment and make it more conducive keeping in view the health and safety of workers;
- develop working cultures incorporating the essential value systems and quality management practices to improve OHS;

The science and practice of occupational health involve several other disciplines, like occupational medicine, nursing, ergonomics, psychology, hygiene, safety, and others. Occupational health is a diverse science that involves the participation of occupational health professional engineers, environmental health practitioners, chemists, toxicologists, doctors, nurses, safety professionals, etc. According to the World Health Organization (1995), occupational safety and health can be defined as:

> "… a multidisciplinary activity aiming at protection and promotion of the health of workers by removing occupational factors and conditions hazardous to health and safety at workplace and enhancing the physical, mental and social well-being of workers and supporting their development and maintenance of their working capacity, together with their professional and social development at workplace …"

According to the World Health Organization (WHO), occupational health deals with diverse facets of health and safety at workstation and is focused on primary prevention of hazards. Since 1950, the International Labour Organization (ILO) and World Health Organization (WHO) have shared a common definition of occupational health. Later, it was adopted by the joint committee on occupational health at its first session in 1950 and reviewed in 1995. It states that the:

Main focus in occupational health is on three different objectives:

1. the maintenance and promotion of workers' health and working capacity;
2. the improvement of working environment and work to become conducive to safety and health; and
3. development of work organizations and working cultures in a direction which supports health and safety at work and in doing so also promotes a positive social climate and smooth operation and may enhance productivity of the undertakings

The concept of working culture envisioned in this context means a reflection of the essential value systems adopted by the concerned undertaking. Factors affecting occupational health include:

- prevailing infrastructure of health services
- reconnaissance of working environment through epidemiological studies and analysis
- skilled manpower
- type of workplace – small, medium, or large and its location
- workers' participation and proprietors' commitment

2.2 WORKPLACE ENVIRONMENT AND WORKPLACE HAZARDS

The workplace environment, irrespective of the work being undertaken, affects employees' health and safety. Human beings are exposed to harmful hazardous chemicals at the workplace and living environment because of rapid industrialization in the modern world. The workplace environment including physical and chemical agents can cause numerous diseases, together with inadequate breathing capability, inflammatory dermal conditions, psycho-neurological disorders, and neoplastic diseases. In the last few years, disciplines that study the effect of workplace environment on human health have seen rapid development. Still, adequate data to categorize these chemicals based on their physico-chemical and toxic properties are available for only 14 percent of the commonly used compounds. Research in the field of industrial toxicology thus classifies the hazards posed by chemical and physical agents to human health present in the workplace and living environment. Occupational Exposure Limit (OEL) is thus the key standard for assessment of occupational exposure and safe use of chemicals at workplace. No matter how small or large, every proprietor needs to have a safe working environment. This responsibility not only stands as a moral and a legal obligation but also in the context of financial purpose. Over the last few decades, agencies like the Occupational Safety and Health Administration (OSHA) have made considerable progress in workplace safety. The incidence of workplace hazards, accidents, and casualties depends on the nature of work undertaken, for instance, the nature of some industrial setups makes them more susceptible to incidents. Construction activities, for example, account for one in five worker deaths in the private sector, other vulnerable industries being transportation, manufacturing, healthcare, and warehousing.

Whether safety incidents result from falls or overexertion, their expenses and implications are always very high, which is in addition to their probable legal expenses. Safety hazards exist in every workplace, but by identifying workplace hazards, these can be controlled or eliminated. A hazard, in the context of workplace health and safety, is "*any source of potential damage, harm or adverse health effects on something or someone*".

A hazard includes the potential harm or adverse effect to people, to property or equipment, or to the environment while risk is the likelihood of harm or adverse health effect a person is likely to experience when exposed to a hazard. Environmental health refers to regulating health hazards at workplace, which involves assessing an environment to ascertain possible hazardous agents and taking suitable measures for offering protection to the workers.

2.2.1 Characteristics of the Workplace Environment

Characteristics of occupational health at the workplace include:

- Active and functional OHS committee at the workplace
- Health education and safety awareness for the employees
- Management and supervision of hygiene and sanitary facilities among the employees
- Monitoring and control of workplace hazards
- OHS regulations
- Pre-appointment and quarterly health check-ups of employees
- Provision of first aid
- Reporting and maintenance of records and data related to occupational deaths, diseases, injuries, disabilities, hazards, and related preventive measures at the workplace
- Review of health safety of shielding/protective devices

The four basic essentials in an occupational setting are summarized in Table 2.1.

2.2.2 Identifying Safety and Health Hazards

A hazard is something that can cause harm if not controlled, while risk is a combination of the possibility that a specific outcome will occur and the severity of the harm involved. The outcome is the damage that results from an unrestrained hazard. 'Hazard', 'risk', and 'outcome' are used to describe environmental damage or damage to equipment. 'Harm' generally describes the direct or indirect degradation, or the temporary or permanent degradation including physical, mental, or social well-being of employees. Workers can face many health risks in a work environment, including the following:

- Biological Hazards
- Chemical Hazards
- Environmental Hazards
- Ergonomic Hazards
- Physical Hazards
- Safety Hazards

Hazard Identification: Hazard identification is a vital step in the overall risk assessment and risk management process. In this, the individual work hazards are recognized, evaluated, and controlled/eradicated as close to source as cautiously as possible. While technology, resources, social suspense, or supervision calls for transformation, hazard analysis focuses on control more closely toward the source of the hazard. Thus, hazard control is a dynamic program of prevention. Hazard-based plans also have the benefit of not assigning or suggesting that there are '*acceptable risks*' in the workplace.

TABLE 2.1
Basic Essentials in an Occupational Setting

Worker/Employee	Workers, mainly the labourers are at risk of occupational hazards due to: • Low education/literacy rates • Inexperience of work and exposures and insufficient training • Tendency of not complaining about working conditions or exposures • High prevalence of endemic (mainly infections) diseases and malnutrition • Inadequate infrastructure and human resources to diagnose, treat, and prevent occupation-related diseases and injuries • Vulnerable groups including women, and children, who account for a significant part of the workforce in many developing countries, often undertake some of the hazardous work. • Lack of legal protections against child labour • Poor and unhygienic living conditions of workers
Tool/Equipment	• Use of primitive/out-dated tools • Lack of awareness about using modern technology/automated equipment • Inappropriately designed tools, working areas, or work procedures
Process/Technique	• The material used in the process can be potentially toxic/hazardous or harmful • The process can be unsafe/tedious or use may expose the workers to heat/dust/radioactive compounds, etc.
Working Environment (external conditions and influences prevailing at workplace interaction in a working environment)	1. **Man and physical, chemical, and biological agents** a. **Physical agents** (noise, heat, humidity, dust, vibration, electricity or lighting, radiation, etc.) b. **Chemical agents** (chemical dust, mists, fumes, liquids, vapours, gases, dust, etc.) c. **Biological agents** (insects and rodents, microorganisms, poisonous plants and animals) d. **Ergonomic hazards** 2. **Man and machine** (interaction with machinery) • Unguarded machines, protruding and moving parts • Poor electrical and machinery installation of equipment/ machinery • Lack of safety measures • Working for long duration in awkward postures/positions can cause fatigue, backache, diseases of joints and muscles, and impairment of the workers' health and efficiency 3. **Man and Psychosocial Environment** • Type and rhythm of work and work stability • Service conditions and security • Job satisfaction, leadership style • Workers' participation and communication • Motivation and incentives

Occupational Risk Assessment: Occupational safety and health regulation generally calls for a risk assessment to be carried out before making an intervention. This assessment must:

- Identify the hazards
- Ascertain all who are likely to be affected by the hazard and possibly how
- Assess the risk
- Identify and prioritize appropriate control measures

Calculation of risk is based on the probability of the harm being identified and the severity of the magnitude and can be expressed precisely as a quantitative assessment, or qualitatively as an account of the situation by which the harm could arise. The assessment must be recorded and reviewed intermittently and when there is a substantial change to work practices. The assessment must include practical suggestions to control the risk. Once suggested controls are executed, the risk must be re-calculated to ascertain if it has been lowered to a satisfactory level. One of the '*root causes*' of workplace injuries, sicknesses, and happenings is the failure to classify or recognize hazards that are present, or that could have been predicted. A vital component of any efficient safety and health program is a hands-on method to recognize and evaluate such hazards. To identify and assess hazards, proprietor and labour:

- Assemble similar incidents and classify trends in reported injuries, illnesses, and hazards.
- Deliberate on risks linked with emergency or non-routine situations.
- Determine the gravity and probability of events that could result for each recognized hazard, and use this data to line up corrective actions.
- Gather and go through the information about the threats present or expected to be present in the workplace.
- Study injuries, illnesses, incidents, and close calls/near misses to regulate the underlying hazards, their bases, and safety and health program inadequacies.
- Undertake the initial and periodic workplace check-ups of the workplace to recognize new or recurrent hazards.

Some hazards, such as housekeeping and falling hazards can and must be fixed as and when they are recognized. Fixing hazards on the spot stresses the significance of safety and health and takes advantage of a safety management prospect. This requires a series of actions, viz.:

Action 1: Gathering the existing information about workplace hazards, both from internal and external sources

Method: Gather, arrange, and evaluate the data to ascertain the types of hazards present and who is likely to be exposed. Available data at workplace may include:

- Employees' compensation records and reports
- Equipment and machinery operating manuals
- Existing safety and health databases and arrangements
- Feedback from employees, including surveys or minutes of safety and health committee meetings
- Outcomes of job hazard analyses
- Patterns of frequently occurring injuries and illnesses
- Records of previous monitoring, industrial hygiene assessments, and medical examinations
- Registers of previous injuries and illnesses
- Safety Data Sheets (SDS) provided by chemical manufacturers
- Self-inspection reports and inspection reports from insurance companies, government agencies, and consultants

Information about hazards may be available from outside sources, such as:

- Labour unions
- Safety and health consultants
- State and local occupational safety and health committees
- Trade associations
- Worker advocacy groups

Action 2: Inspection of the workplace for safety hazards

Hazards can be introduced over time due to:

- Change in workplaces and procedures
- Decline in housekeeping practices
- Negligence in maintenance
- Worn-out equipment or tools

Frequent inspection of workplace for hazards not only helps in recognizing faults but gives time to efficiently handle the occurrence of incidents.

Method: The handling involves various measures which can be achieved by:

- Conducting regular inspections of all operations, equipment, work areas, and facilities
- Ensuring workers' participation in the inspection team and conversation with them about the hazards pointed out in the reports.
- Undertaking inspections so that these can be verified later and risky situations are amended
- Audio-visual documentation of problem areas to enable subsequent conversation and brainstorming on controlling them
- Covering all areas and activities in inspections, for example, storage and warehousing, facility and equipment repairs, procurement, and the activities of on-site contractors, subcontractors, and temporary workers

- Frequently inspecting transportation vehicles
- Using checklists that highlight things to look for; each workplace will have its own list with regard to:
  - Electrical hazards
  - Equipment operation and maintenance
  - Ergonomic complications
  - Fire safety
  - General housekeeping
  - Lack of emergency measures
  - Slip, trip, and fall hazards
  - Work organization and process flow (including staffing and scheduling)
  - Work practices
  - Workplace violence
- Seeking the input of workers and evaluating the planned changes for potential hazards and related risks before changing the operations, workstations, or workflow
- Seeking the input of workers before making major organizational changes or introducing new equipment, materials, or processes

Action 3: Identification of potential health hazards

Identifying employees' exposure to health hazards is more difficult than recognizing physical safety hazards, for example, gases and vapours may be invisible, often without any odour, and may not have an instantaneously perceptible harmful health effect. Health hazards include:

- Biological hazards (infectious diseases)
- Chemical hazards (solvents, adhesives, paints, toxic dusts, etc.)
- Ergonomic risk factors (heavy lifting, repetitive motions, vibration, etc.)
- Physical hazards (noise, radiation, heat, etc.)

Reviewing workers' medical records can be useful in identifying health hazards linked with workplace exposures.

Method: It involves:

- Identifying chemical hazards (reviewing the SDS and product labels to identify the workplace chemicals that have low exposure limits, are highly volatile, or are used in large quantities and identifying activities that may result in exposure to chemicals)
- Identifying physical hazards (detect any exposure to excessive noise, elevated heat, or sources of radiation)
- Identifying biological hazards (determining if the workers are exposed to sources of infectious diseases, moulds, toxic or poisonous plants, or animal materials capable of causing allergic reactions)
- Identifying ergonomic risk factors (grouping work activities that necessitate heavy lifting, work above shoulder height, repetitive motions, etc.)

- Conducting quantitative exposure assessments
- Periodically reviewing medical records to identify cases of musculoskeletal injuries, dermatitis, hearing loss, or lung disease linked with workplace exposures

Action 4: Conducting incident investigations

Workplace incidents, including injuries, illnesses, close calls/near miss, and reports of other concerns give a clear picture of site of hazards. By carefully examining the incidents and reports, hazards that can cause future harm be identified. The purpose of an exploration should be to identify the root cause of the incident to prevent future incidences.

Method: It involves a series of protocols like:

- Developing a well-defined and clear-cut plan and procedure for undertaking enquiry of occurrence of event, so that an investigation can start instantaneously when an event happens and the plan must cover items such as:
  - Who will be involved
  - Lines of communication
  - Desirable materials, equipment, and supplies
  - Describing forms and templates
- Training of the investigation teams on investigation techniques, highlighting fairness and impartiality during the course of the investigation
- Conducting investigations with a trained team including representatives of both management and workers
- Investigating close calls/near misses
- Identifying and analysing the root causes to focus on causal faults that permitted the incidents to occur
- Communicate the outcomes of the investigation to managers, supervisors, and workers to avoid relapse

Action 5: Identifying hazards linked with emergency and non-routine situations

Non-routine or infrequent works, including maintenance and start-up/shutdown activities, also cause potential hazards. Plans and procedures must be evolved for reacting suitably and safely to hazards linked to probable emergency scenarios and non-routine circumstances.

Method: Probable emergency scenarios and non-routine tasks must be identified, in view of the types of material and equipment in use and the site. Following situations may be predictable:

- Chemical emissions
- Disease occurrences
- Fires and explosions
- Medical emergencies
- Natural disasters

- Non-routine tasks
- Spilling of hazardous material
- Structural collapse
- Violence at workplace
- Weather emergencies

Action 6: Describing the type of identified hazards, and classifying interim control measures

The next step is to evaluate and comprehend the identified hazards and the kinds of incidents that could result from exposure to those hazards. This data can be used to develop interim controls and to prioritize hazards for permanent control.

Method: This involves:

- Assessment of each hazard by taking into account the severity of potential consequences, the probability that an event or exposure will occur, and the number of workers who might be exposed.
- Using temporary controlling measures to safeguard workers till permanent solutions can be executed.
- Prioritizing hazards so that those posing the greatest threat are addressed earliest.

2.2.3 Accountability for Safety and Health Hazards

People accountable for categorizing and improving health and safety hazards:

- Authorized personnel
- Contractors
- Employers
- Owners
- Self-employers
- Supervisors
- Suppliers
- Workers

Occupational health team consists of:

- Ergonomist
- Health educator
- Industrial psychologist
- Industrial toxicologist
- Occupational health epidemiologist
- Occupational health nurse
- Occupational health physician
- Occupational hygienist
- Occupational therapist

- Physiotherapist
- Safety engineer

Ergonomist is one who:

- designs the work and workplace to fit the worker
- deals with designing and changing the workplace to ensure that employees are not injured or catch diseases while working

Hygienist is:

- responsible for recognizing, evaluating, and controlling health hazards at workplace
- one who examines the working environment and work activities

Components of Occupational Health

- Educational rehabilitation
- First aid education
- First aid treatment in emergency
- Health counseling
- Health education
- Medical examination
- Medical rehabilitation
- Medical treatment
- Mental and physical health
- Periodic medical examination
- Pre-employment examination
- Rehabilitation program
- Social rehabilitation
- Special medical examination
- Stress management
- Vocational rehabilitation

BIBLIOGRAPHY

Aburumman, M., Newnam, S. and Fildes, B. (2019) Evaluating the effectiveness of workplace interventions in improving safety culture: A systematic review. Safety Science 115:376–392.

Alli, B. (2001) Fundamental Principles of Occupational Health and Safety. Geneva: International Labour Organization.

Bayley, J. (1991) Health and safety at work. British Dental Journal 170(10):364–365.

Christian, M. S., Bradley, J. C., Wallace, J. C. and Burke, M. J. (2009) Workplace safety: A meta-analysis of the roles of person and situation factors. Journal of Applied Psychology 94(5):1103–1127.

Cutler, R. (1991) Health and safety at work. British Dental Journal 170(7):251.

Forst, L., Nickels, L. and Conroy, L. (2009) The WHO modules in occupational safety and health: Training for prevention. Public Health Reports 124(1):169–176.
Gunningham, N. (2005) Safety, regulation and the mines inspectorate: Lessons from Western Australia. Journal of Occupational Health and Safety 21(4):299.
Hernberg, S. (1992) Introduction to Occupational Epidemiology. Philadelphia: Lewis Publishers.
IAEA, ILO, WHO. (1998) Health surveillance of persons occupationally exposed to ionizing radiation: Guidance for occupational physicians, Safety Reports Series No. 5. Vienna: IAEA, ILO, WHO.
IAEA. (1999) Assessment of occupational exposure due to external sources of radiation IAEA Safety Standards, Series No. RS-G-1.3. Vienna: International Atomic Energy Agency.
IAEA. (1999) Occupational radiation protection IAEA Safety Standards, Series No. RS-G-1.1. Vienna: International Atomic Energy Agency.
ILO. (2001) Ambient Factors in the Workplace: An ILO code of practice. Geneva: International Labour Organization.
Jonathan, G. K. and Rosemary, W. M. (2016) Maintaining health and safety at workplace: Employee and employer's role in ensuring a safe working environment. International University Journal of Education and Practice 7(29):1–7.
Levy, B. S. and Wegman, D. H. (1994) Occupational Health: Recognizing and Preventing Work-Related Disease. Boston: Little Brown.
Magalhães, L. M. C. A. *et al.* (2022) A study on occupational health and safety. BMC Public Health 22:2186.
Nichols, T. (1998) Health and safety at work. Work, Employment & Society 12(2):367–374.
Qasim, M., Bashir, A., Shan, A. and Anees, M. M. (2014) Concept of occupational health and safety and evaluation of awareness level among employees. World Applied Sciences Journal 32(5):904–909.
Rosenstock, L. and Cullen, M. R. (1994) Textbook of Clinical Occupational and Environmental Medicine. Philadelphia: Saunders.
Sánchez, F. A. S., Peláez, G. I. C. and Alí, J. C. S. (2017) Occupational safety and health in construction: A review of applications and trends. Industrial Health 55:210–218.
Scott, R. M. (2020) Chemical Hazards in the Workplace (e-book). Boca Raton: CRC Press.
Spurlock, B. (2017) Physical Hazards of the Workplace. Boca Raton: CRC Press.
Stout, N. A. and Linn, H. I. (2002) Occupational injury prevention research: Progress and priorities. Injury Prevention 8:9–14.
Suparna, N. S. and Jaiswal, A. (2021) The occupational health and safety. Anthropo-Indialogs 1(3):261–269.
WHO. (2005) Occupational Health. Geneva, Switzerland: World Health Organization.
WHO. (2011) Global Status Report on Non-communicable Diseases 2010. Geneva: World Health Organization.
Wilson, H. G. E. and Agius, R. M. (1994) Health and safety at work. BMJ 309(6948):198–199.

3 Workplace Hazards

Biological

"Safety is not a gadget, but a state of mind"

– Eleanor Everet

FACT FILE

- Bacteria, viruses, parasites, fungi, and prions in food are the main biological hazards that severely affect humans and animal health
- Workers in the health and community services, viz. agriculture, forestry, and fishing industries were most likely to report exposure to biological hazards
- The COVID-19 pandemic has highlighted the potentially shocking global impact of uncontrolled biological hazards
- Diseases, such as Severe Acute Respiratory Syndrome (SARS), influenza A (H_1N_1), and Ebola fever are of international concern
- Exposure to viruses that cause contagious diseases is but one of the numerous biological hazards workers are exposed to
- In workplaces such as hospitals and laboratories, cattle-producing factories, sewage maintenance facilities, waste collection, and many other activities, workers are exposed to biological hazards including bacteria, viruses, parasites, fungi, prions, DNA material, bodily fluids as well as other microorganisms and their associated allergens and toxins
- Zoonotic diseases originate from human interaction with animals
- There are over 200 types of zoonoses
- Zoonoses can also cause disruptions in the production and trade of animal products for food and other uses
- The COVID-19 pandemic was caused by the zoonotic virus SARS-CoV-2
- The spread of diseases is increased by global mobility and interaction and is driven by globalized movements of goods and persons including tourism, and business-related travels
- Biotechnology, genetic engineering, and infection control also affect the development of biological hazards
- Genetically modified plants or animals developed for use in agriculture, horticulture, food industry, medical research, and the pharmaceutical industry. Though genetically modified organisms (GMOs) have the possibility of human development, consideration is essential, from a legal perspective, to provide guidance on the impact of GMOs on human health particularly the workers who are directly exposed to them

DOI: 10.1201/9781003464785-3

3.1 INTRODUCTION

Each day, the employees came across various workplace hazards. Among various hazards, biological hazards present a severe and serious threat to the safety and health of workers. It is vital to recognize what biological hazards are, how they are categorized, and what should be done to mitigate the linked risks to help in safeguarding oneself from probable exposure to biological hazards. Workplace biological hazards, also known as workplace bio-hazards, are caused by biological agents/substances or organisms that endanger employees' health. These hazards can be caused by bacteria, viruses, fungi (including yeasts and moulds), internal human parasites (endo-parasites), and toxins, which pose threats to the health of other living organisms, generally humans and animals. Workers are exposed to biological agents at the workplace. Biological agents can cause various illnesses, from minor skin infections to life-threatening diseases. The incidence of biological hazards is usually more in workplaces, including healthcare facilities, laboratories, and industrial setups. Employees can be exposed to biological hazards through contact with infected animals or people. There are many agents, substances, and settings which can create biological hazards in working environment and there are different methods of determining them. Biological agents are extensively distributed in the natural environment and consequently found in many work sectors. The majority of these agents are not dangerous, but some may have the potential to cause illness.

Types of Biological Hazards: Alike other workplace hazards, biological hazards have the capacity to harm and infect workers, mainly those who are directly exposed to them. While most bio-hazards often come from microbes, they are categorized into four major types:

Biological Agents: This group includes bacteria, viruses, parasites, and fungi (such as yeasts and moulds). These are commonly considered nontoxic, undamaging, and non-detrimental if kept under controlled conditions, but once released some of them may cause serious hazards and diseases in animals or human beings, such as the COVID-19 virus.

Bio-toxins: These include a group of substances with a biological origin which are toxic and poisonous to humans. Bio-toxins are produced by plants, bacteria, insects, or certain animals. Constant exposure to bio-toxins may cause a series of inflammation in the body.

Blood and Blood Products: These include contaminated blood products such as RBCs, WBCs, plasma, tissues, and platelets which may be hazardous if not properly handled.

Environmental Samples: These usually refer to plants, soil, or water that possibly contain biological agents and bio-toxins.

3.1.1 Types of Exposure

In workplaces, exposure to biological agents can be:

- deliberate, where the worker works directly with them, maybe, in a laboratory or research facility, or

- unintended, where the worker is exposed to the biological agent because of the work they perform, for instance, a healthcare worker is exposed to a blood-borne virus, a laundry worker who gets a needle stick injury, or a farmer is exposed to livestock disease that can also have an impact on humans (a zoonosis).

Biological agents are categorized into the following risk groups. The grouping system is based on the fact that the agent:

- is pathogenic to human beings
- is a threat to employees
- is communicable to the community and there is effective therapy/ medication or prophylactic measures are available

Risks of Biological Hazards: To help organizations, Environment, Health, and Safety (EHS) managers and workers properly identify the potential threats or risks that the various types of biological hazards pose, a system of risk group classification for biological agents is established. This system is also used as a guide in implementing effective measures based on the degree of risk. According to the World Health Organization, Risk Groups I to IV pertain to the following:

- **Risk Group I (low to no individual or community risk):** Biological agents or organisms that are unlikely to cause diseases in healthy human beings or animals
- **Risk Group II (moderate individual risk, low community risk):** This group includes pathogens that probably cause diseases among human beings or animals but have minimal hazards among the workers, community, or the environment
- **Risk Group III (high individual risk, low community risk):** This group includes pathogens causing serious diseases among human beings or animals that don't normally spread from one infected individual to another, and for this group preventive and treatment measures may be accessible
- **Risk Group IV (high individual and community risk):** This group includes pathogens that are directly or indirectly transmissible and cause serious ailments among human beings or animals and for this group preventive and treatment measures may not be accessible

3.1.2 Effects of Biological Agents

Risk Group Categorization: Tables 3.1 to 3.6 classify occupational infections into six categories:

Since biological agents are usually invisible, it is often difficult to assume the threats they can pose. The worker may be harmed by after:

- an allergic reaction to the biological agent or toxins it produces

TABLE 3.1
Contact with Infected Living Animal

Professions	Cause of Contact	Infections and Diseases
• Animal breeder/caretaker/scientist • Farmer/farm worker	Involved in handling infected domestic animals (probably inhalation or percutaneous exposure)	Anthrax, Brucellosis, Hendra and Nipah viral diseases, Influenza, Leptospirosis, Plague, Q fever, Vesicular stomatitis fever
• Laboratory attendant/assistant • Veterinary personnel	Bite or scratch by infected dog or cat	Brucellosis, Capnocytophaga infection, Cat scratch fever, Pasteurellosis, Plague, Rabies, Tularemia
• Animal breeder/caretaker/scientist • Laboratory attendant/assistant • Veterinary personnel • Poultry farmer/worker	Involved in handling chickens or birds	*Campylobacter enteritis*, Influenza, Psittacosis, Salmonellosis
• Farmer • Hunter • Veterinary personnel • Wildlife biologist	Bite by skunk, raccoon, bat, fox, or other carnivore	Rabies
• Farmer • Hunter	Bite by rodents	Monkeypox, Plague, Rat bite fever
• Veterinary personnel • Wildlife biologist	Involved in handling infected rodents (probably inhalation or percutaneous exposure)	Hantavirus infection, Lassa fever, Leptospirosis, Lymphocytic choriomeningitis (LCM), Monkeypox, Plague
• Laboratory attendant/assistant	Involved in handling infected laboratory rats	Hantavirus infection, LCM, Rat bite fever
• Veterinary personnel	Handling infected macaque monkeys	B-virus infection

TABLE 3.2
Contact with Contaminated Animal Product

Professions	Cause of Contact	Infections and Diseases
• Animal breeder/caretaker/scientist • Farmer/farm worker • Laboratory attendant/assistant • Butcher/hunter/slaughterer • Farmer • Meat packer • Veterinary personnel	Involved in handling infected animal carcasses or placental tissues	Anthrax, Brucellosis, Glanders, Hendra and Nipah viral diseases, Leptospirosis, Plague, Psittacosis, Q fever, Rift Valley fever, Tularemia
• Grader/sorter • Consignment supervisor • Packer	Involved in handling raw goat hair, wool, or hides from endemic area	Anthrax

TABLE 3.3
Contact with Ticks, Fleas, or Mites

Professions	Cause of Contact	Infections and Diseases
• Farmer/farm worker • Forester • Hunter • Landscaper • Logging worker	Working in tick-infested area	Babesiosis, Lyme disease, Powassan virus encephalitis, Relapsing fever, Rocky Mountain spotted fever, Tick paralysis, Tularemia
• Building cleaning worker • Pest control worker	Working in building infested with fleas or mites of rodents	Murine typhus, Plague, Rickettsia pox
• Hunter • Worker	Working in mite-infested area	Scrub typhus

- being exposed to toxins produced by the biological agent, or
- getting infected by a biological agent

Biological agents have the ability to multiply quickly, require negligible resources to live, and can infect even in minute doses. Biological hazards are of organic origin or caused by biological vectors, including pathogenic microbes, toxins, and bioactive substances, which may pose a risk to animals, including livestock, and to plants. The impact of biological hazards manifests in the form of economic and environmental losses. The following outbreaks, epidemics, or pandemics are caused by biological hazards:

- Ebola virus disease outbreak in West Africa in 2013–2016, the largest epidemic of its kind to date in the populations of Guinea, Liberia, and Sierra Leone

TABLE 3.4
Contact with Human or Animal Waste

Professions	Cause of Contact	Infections and Diseases
• Childcare worker • Laboratory attendant/assistant • Veterinary personnel	Involved in taking care of children or primates infected with Hepatitis A virus	Hepatitis A
• Farmer/farm worker • Septic tank worker	Involved in swimming in contaminated water (due to percutaneous exposure)	Leptospirosis, Schistosomiasis
• Livestock/cattle supervisor • Childcare worker	Involved in taking care of children or animals infected with cryptosporidiosis	Cryptosporidiosis
• Animal breeder/caretaker/scientist • Farmer/farm worker • Laboratory attendant/assistant • Veterinary personnel	Dog or cat contact (faecal-oral)	Campylobacter enteritis, Echinococcosis, Hymenolepsis nana infection, Salmonellosis, Yersinosis

TABLE 3.5
Contact with Infected Patient or Blood

Professions	Cause of Contact	Infections and Diseases
• Dental worker • Healthcare worker	Involved in handling contaminated needles or surgical instruments	AIDS, Ebola – Marburg, Hepatitis B, Hepatitis C, Lassa fever
• Healthcare worker	Involved in taking care of sick patients (droplet/airborne pathogens)	Adenovirus, Coronavirus infection, Haemorrhagic fever, Diphtheria, Ebola, Influenza, Measles, Monkeypox, Mumps, Mycoplasma infection, Parvor-Virus, Pertussis, Rubella, Tuberculosis
	Involved in taking care of sick patients (blood-borne pathogens)	AIDS, Haemorrhagic fever, Ebola, Hepatitis B, Hepatitis C, Lassa fever

- Outbreak of Zika virus infection in the Americas and the Pacific region
- Epidemic of yellow fever in Angola, the Democratic Republic of Congo, and Uganda in 2016
- The COVID-19 pandemic in the year 2020 throughout the world taking the lives of lakhs of people

Risk assessment of biological hazards is challenging due to their unique characteristics:

Agent diversity: Biological hazards range from microbes such as bacteria or viruses to toxins to insect infestations, which can be transmitted to human beings from the environment, animals, plants, and other humans.

TABLE 3.6
Contact with Pathogen-infected Dust

Professions	Cause of Contact	Infections and Diseases
• Building cleaning worker • Construction worker • Farmer/farm worker • Groundskeeper • Heating and AC worker • Hunter • Pest control worker • Repair worker • Wildlife biologist	Dust containing excreta of rodents	Hantavirus infection, Leptospirosis, Rat bite fever
• Painter • Construction worker • Demolition worker • Farmer/farm worker • Gardener • AC worker	Dust released from bird nestles, chicken cages, or bat-inhabited fissures in endemic area	Histoplasmosis
• Archaeologist • Demolition worker • Farmer • Hunter	Excavated soil in endemic area	Blastomycosis, Coccidioidomycosis, Histoplasmosis

Transmission Route: This includes:

- Airborne transmission
- Ingestion
- Absorption (through the skin, eyes, mucous membranes, wounds)
- Animal vectors (e.g. mosquitos or ticks)
- Bodily fluids (e.g. blood, mother to child transmission, sexual transmission)

Pathogenicity and virulence: Bio-hazards can cause severe diseases even in extremely low concentration and can reproduce rapidly once they enter the body of the host.

Hazard identification: Since microbes are not visible to the naked eye, they are not easily detectable. They can be identified using epidemiological information based on clinical signs and symptoms. Therefore, these require specific diagnosis methods, like polymerase chain reaction (PCR), microbial cultures, and whole genome sequencing.

Prevalent diseases with probability for epidemic transmission: Biological hazards exist in the community, i.e. they are widespread and usually pose low risk when the population is generally resistant. The risk may change when calamities or crises befall, worsening the situations favourable for transmission of disease, or when individuals travel from disease-free areas to endemic regions usually lacking resistance, making them vulnerable to infection and transmission of disease. Biological hazards, which are not widespread also, pose a threat when they are initiated in a new host community with lacking immunity.

Sensitivity to climate, ecological, or land use changes: Biological hazards, mainly zoonosis and vector-borne diseases such as malaria, dengue, Zika, and Ebola, may increase in incidence, lethality, or change topographical distribution or seasonal patterns. This is due to weather sensitivity, ecological or land use transformations, or facilitated through changes in ecosystems due to anthropogenic activities, consequently changing human exposure and vulnerability to these hazards. Approximately 75 percent of incipient infectious human diseases that have grown after exposure to zoonotic pathogens demand risk assessment for health-related risks after the interaction between animals, humans, and ecosystems.

3.2 BIOLOGICAL RISK MANAGEMENT AT WORKPLACE

Biological risk management system must be erected on the concept of constant improvement through a cycle of planning, implementing, reviewing, and improving the processes and actions that an organization undertakes to realize its objectives.

Identification and Risk Assessment: The identification of biological hazards at the workplace must consider the:

- modes of transmission (direct or indirect contact, aerosols, water, surfaces, vectors, food);
- pathological mechanisms;
- previous injuries and illness;
- the circumstances or events with the possibility of giving rise to injury or illness;
- the nature of potential injury or illness related to the circumstances;
- those expected to be affected (viz. young/older worker, temporary worker, pregnant worker); and
- transmission entry/routes of exposure (viz. inhalation, ingestion, dermal, etc.)

Risk Assessment: It is a process which determines the level of possibility of injury or disease linked with each recognized hazard for regulating the same. In establishing the risk level, special consideration must be given to factors such as sex, age, infirmity, the health status of worker, and comorbidities. Undertaking biological risk assessment involves five steps:

- documentation of biological hazards;
- detection of who might be affected and how;
- estimation of the biological risks and methods of controlling them;
- documenting the outcome of the biological risk assessment and fixing the priorities for enhancement; and
- re-evaluating and apprising the biological risk assessment, as required

The assessment of biological risks must categorize each hazard based on its:

- accessibility and efficacy of protective methods
- accessibility of efficient control measures
- availability and efficacy of medical treatments
- incidence of a pathogen
- mode of spread
- possibility of causing harm (contamination, allergy, toxicity)
- probable aerosol generation
- reservoir of the agent
- seriousness of its probable harm
- stability in the environment
- transmissibility within a population

The identification of employees who can be harmed when exposed to biological hazards must take into account:

- antigen or antibody test results of worker
- medical history of worker
- health status of worker
- use and availability of prophylactic treatments
- vaccination status of worker; and
- underlying conditions

Risk assessment methods must be chosen based on a classification of the concerned hazards. Priorities for action must be evolved based on the probability and gravity of harm that the biological hazards can cause.

Evaluating the threat of biological hazards: Methods for evaluating the threats of biological hazards vary according to the objective of the evaluation:

- Strategic Risk Assessment is used for risk management planning with an emphasis on prevention and preparedness measures, capacity development, and medium- to longer-term risk monitoring and evaluation.
- Rapid Risk Assessment is used to evaluate, regulate, and control the level of risk linked with perceived events and to consequently define response mediations.
- Post-event evaluation is used for recovery planning, updating, and firming the inclusive risk management system.

3.2.1 Pre-event: Strategic Risk Assessment

These assessments are used for:

- Risk management planning with a focus on prevention and preparedness
- Capacity building before the occurrence of any event
- Medium- to longer-term risk monitoring and evaluation

- Tracking changes in risk over time
- Catalysing the planned actions to lessen the level of risk and effects on health outcomes taking into account the estimation of the hazard, exposure, susceptibilities and capabilities

While addressing the risks of biological hazards, the term vulnerability means the risk factors that exist in exposed populations, such as:

- Burden of endemic diseases
- Living conditions (e.g. congestion)
- Environment (e.g. congenial environment for development of the pathogen)
- Demographics (e.g. age or gender)
- Accessibility of healthcare services to the populations
- Degree of resilience of the healthcare systems

Quantitative Microbiological Risk Assessment (QMRA): QMRA is an important example of a strategic risk assessment method for assessment of biological hazard evolved for prevention and mitigation of risks, and includes:

- detecting the features of the pathogen/microbial agent (i.e. fatality ratio, transmission route, incubation times)
- human diseases linked with the specific microorganism

QMRA assesses the dose of the pathogen that an individual consumes, breathes in, or comes in contact with. It also needs information on the concentration of pathogen in the source, route of transmission, and exposure timing. Different approaches are used for defining the status of risks linked with biological hazards, comprising multi-criteria decision analysis (MCDA) and burden of diseases. These methods allow for better risk ranking and scheduling of public health alertness.

STAR Approach: World Health Organization (WHO) STAR approach to strategic risk assessment empowers nations to include an evidence-based approach to strategic risk assessments. The STAR approach is evolved to:

- Involve multi-sectoral stakeholders in risk assessment developed for hazards affecting public health;
- Offer a systematic, transparent, and evidence-based approach to identify, rank, and classify priority hazards by level of risk;
- Define the level of national preparedness and promptness essential to alleviate each hazard and its risk

Multi-Criteria Decision Analysis (MCDA): It is a randomized method in which several standards with their intensities are categorized in line with the outcome of interest. Conditions may include information on epidemiology, economics, and data on perception of the diseases. The conditions can have equal or different weights depending on their relative significance for the result. These data can be gathered from literature, databanks from official sources, and incidence studies. The Global Burden of Disease (GBD) estimations make available inclusive and analogous evaluation of mortality and loss of health due to diseases, injuries, and risk factors. The estimates provide an overview of the changing health challenges people are facing across the world.

Rapid Risk Assessment: In case of incidence of any event, the risk level posed by the event is assessed through rapid risk assessments to give early warning and response measures. The risk assessment of communicable diseases takes into account the likelihood of transmission of disease in the population and severity of the disease, and the setting in which the disease occurs. The initial rapid risk assessment must be carried out within a short duration. The assessment must be undertaken in the initial stages of an event, and if possible should be produced within 24 to 48 hours. The level of risk must be re-assessed based on evolving information on the event and disease pattern. Risk assessment helps in:

- determining whether a response is specified
- the design, and range of control measures
- the necessity, and extent of the response
- wider implications and management of the incident

It is important that during risk assessment the following is available to the team:

- A repository of events that occurred in the past
- Approaches for rapid literature review
- Evidence-based protocols
- List of specialists consulted
- Protocols for recognizing sources of important information for rapid risk assessment

3.2.2 Preventive and Control Measures

The measures must be executed in line with the following principles:

Biological Control (prevent and reduce exposure potentials and their magnitudes by using weakened, substitute organisms or procedures that can incapacitate the biological agent, resulting in reduced replication, infectivity, transmissibility, and virulence)

Work Limitations (confiding the number of workers exposed as low as possible by restraining the workload and restricting work in risk areas)

Protection during Working (minimizing exposure by imposing safe working systems viz. wearing PPE, preventing aerosol generation, training, etc.).

Physical Control (providing extra protection physical barriers for escaping from biological agents, including doors, biological safety cabinets, air filtration systems, wastewater management systems, etc.) Primary barriers minimalize occupational exposure by controlling the transmission. Secondary barriers offer additional control, mostly for evading from biological agents when primary barriers fail.

Hazard Minimization (undertaking activities to decrease the magnitudes of exposure, including emergency measures, contingency policies, health and medical surveillance, or vaccinations to lessen the magnitude of accidental exposure).

The elimination of biological hazards can be realized through:

- cleanliness of buildings, workspaces, and housing
- decontamination of potential sources
- delivery of safe water supplies
- dressing of open wounds
- permutation of disease-eradication methods
- suitable dumping of human and animal waste

Risk Communication: It must be undertaken in an authentic way to convey reliable information so as to avoid misunderstanding. The information to be passed must be comprehensible and clear both for employers and workers. It must be in language selected keeping in view the literacy level of workers and must be beneficial to execute as an effective management system.

Health Surveillance of Workers: Surveillance must be undertaken with a purpose of primary prevention of occupational and work-related injuries, ill health and diseases under controlled conditions. The surveillance must be appropriate to the occupational risks posed by biological hazards. The health surveillance must be done keeping in view the concerned safeguards. The surveillance should be free of charge and must be done during working hours.

Training and Dissemination of Information: Information, instruction, and training must be organized and provided to all workers to make them understand the:

- potential exposure routes of biological hazards at the workplace
- health impacts of biological hazards
- mode of transmission
- symptoms and treatment
- prevention and control of exposure

Individuals who are likely to be affected must receive necessary and suitable information, instruction, and training about the biological hazards. The workers should be properly supervised during the work for use of correct PPE. Worker training must be provided according to the guidance or standards prescribed by the competent authority with regard to biological hazards. Wherever applicable, a special training must be organized for migrant workers. Training must be organized during working hours.

3.2.3 Enquiry of Occupational Accidents and Diseases

After an incidence of occupational accident or disease attributable to biological hazards, an enquiry of its origin and basic reasons must be carried out to find any failures in prevailing prevention and control measures against biological risks at the workplace. The competent authority must hold investigations into cases of dangerous occurrences that appear to reflect serious situations in terms of real or potential risk to employees or the community. The competent authority must take action to prevent a recurrence. The employer must confirm that preparations are ready while undertaking investigation of hazardous occupational accidents and diseases due to biological hazards. The employer should confirm that a competent person is identified to carry out such investigations.

The results of investigations must be communicated to the safety and health committee and the committee must make appropriate suggestions. The results of investigations should be communicated for corrective actions. Epidemiological surveillance and record-keeping must always be ready. Records of occupational accidents and diseases should include:

- action taken to avoid a reappearance; and
- efficiency of the measures taken
- methods for dealing with hazardous incidences, occupational accidents, and diseases
- safety and health problems after exposure to biological agents at the workplace
- sex and age information of workers who might have been exposed
- the causal biological agents
- the mode(s) of transmission of the biological or toxic agent
- the source and site of exposure

Documenting and Notifying Occupational Accidents and Diseases

The competent authority must have a system of notifying the information on occupational accidents, injuries, and diseases. The reporting, recording, notifying, and investigation of occupational accidents, and diseases are necessary for preventing exposure from biological hazards and must be undertaken to:

- categorize safety and health complications arising from exposure to biological agents at the workplace;
- develop efficient and comprehensive approaches for dealing with occupational accidents and diseases;
- explain urgencies for taking action;
- identify probable gaps in legislation and regulations;
- monitor enhancements over time
- provide reliable information on occupational accidents and diseases; and
- supervise the efficiency of measures taken to safeguard adequate safety and health

Preparedness and Response: In the last few decades, the world has seen a variety of emergencies linked with biological hazards, with outbreaks of infectious diseases, for instance, Severe Acute Respiratory Syndrome (SARS), H1N1 influenza, Ebola virus, Zika virus, and COVID-19. Furthermore, pandemics can cause secondary incidents and emergencies at workplaces, as demonstrated by the microbial contamination of workplaces. Climate change, rapid urbanization, and changing land use patterns have increased the threats of emergence of biological hazards and infectious disease at workplace. Temperature rise has amplified the transmission and spread of vector-borne diseases. Emergency preparedness and response measures must be instituted, regularly reviewed, and sustained at work-stations. These arrangements must identify the probability of events, emergencies and outbreaks resulting from biological hazards. Provisions should be made in line with the location and environment of the workplace, and nature of activities. Organizations must develop an emergency action or response plan that takes into consideration the nature of incidents, emergencies, and outbreaks, key responders and their accountabilities, and must:

- confirm that the required information, communication, and coordination are provided to safeguard all people in the incident of emergency or outbreak;
- make available information and communicate with competent authorities, community, and emergency response services; and
- provide relevant information, instruction, and training to all workers at the workplace

Emergency preparedness and response arrangements must be instituted by the company with the help of other employers, workers, and external emergency services. The emergency response plan must be developed locally for each workplace. Alliance with public health, occupational health, veterinary health, and other partners is important for preparedness and response to emergencies including biological hazards, including outbreaks, epidemics, and pandemics. Occupational health service providers must be trained in potential biological hazards in both workplaces and communities. The following steps are evolved to prepare for and manage outbreaks at workplaces:

- identification of biological hazards and
- identification of eradication or prevention measures by immunization;
- early detection of cases of infectious or non-infectious diseases caused by biohazards
- quick reporting of cases through established reporting systems through effective communication
- getting expert advice and support, if required;
- executing a locally and nationally corresponding support system; and
- partnership on research into methods of prevention, treatment and hazard control of prevailing biological hazards

Biological agent outbreak preparedness and response plans must be organized within the framework of analysis focusing on equity and inclusion, according to prevailing human rights frameworks (Table 3.7).

TABLE 3.7
Possible Biological Hazards Associated with Work Activities

List of Activities at Workplace	Possible Hazards and Risks
Food production units	• Allergies caused by moulds/yeasts, bacteria, and mites; • Dust of grains, milk powder, flour contaminated with biological agents; and • Toxins such as botulinus toxins or aflatoxins.
Agriculture, forestry, horticulture, food and fodder production	• Bacteria, fungi, mites, and viruses transferred from animals, parasites, and ticks; • Respiratory problems due to microbes and mites in organic dusts of grain, milk powder, flour, and spices; • Specific allergic diseases for instance farmer's lung and bird breeder's lung; and • Specific risks, such as green tobacco sickness, monkey fever, bites, stings, and venom.
Healthcare and community services	• Several viral and bacterial infections such as HIV, hepatitis, or tuberculosis; and • Sharp and needle stick injuries.
Laboratory	• Infections and allergies caused by handling microorganisms and cell cultures, especially of human tissues; and • Accidental spills and needle stick injuries.
Metal-processing, wood processing, and mining industry	• Skin problems due to bacteria and bronchial asthma due to moulds/yeasts in circulating fluids used in industrial processes such as grinding, fluids used in pulp factories, and metal- and stone-cutting fluids.
Refuse disposal plants, sewage purification installations	• Infections and allergies caused by organic components of bio-wastes, including bacteria, fungi, and their spores and mycotoxins, viruses and prions, parasites, and vector-borne diseases.
Air conditioning systems and high humidity (for example, textile, print, and paper production industry)	• Allergies and respiratory disorders due to moulds/yeasts, Legionella
Archives, museums, libraries	• Moulds/yeasts and bacteria causing allergies and respiratory disorders
Building and construction industry, processing of natural materials	• Moulds and bacteria due to deterioration of building materials

BIBLIOGRAPHY

(2012) Rapid Risk Assessment of Acute Public 14 Health Events. Available from http://apps.who.int/iris/bitstream/10665/70810/1/WHO_HSE_GAR_ARO_2012.1_eng.pdf.

(2015) European Centre for Disease Prevention and Control Burden of Communicable Disease in Europe (BCoDE) toolkit. Version 1.4. Stockholm: ECDC.

(2015) Report of the Ebola Interim Assessment Panel. Available from www.who.int/csr/resources/publications/ebola/report-by-panel.pdf.

(2017) Words into Action Guidelines: National Disaster Risk Assessment Hazard Specific Risk Assessment 5. Biological Hazards Risk Assessment. UNISDR.
Bayley, J. (1991) Health and safety at work. British Dental Journal 170(10):364–365.
Cutler, R. (1991) Health and safety at work. British Dental Journal 170(7).
Dutkiewicz, J., Cisak, E., Sroka, J., Wójcik-Fatla, A. and Zając, V. (2011) Biological agents as occupational hazards—selected issues. Ann Agric Environ Med. 18:286–293.
Hernberg, S. (1992) Introduction to Occupational Epidemiology. Philadelphia: Lewis Publishers.
Jones, A. (2021) Biological Hazards. In The Core Body of Knowledge for Generalist OHS Professionals. 2nd Ed. Tullamarine, VIC: Australian Institute of Health and Safety.
Kyung, R. and Cheol-Hong, L. (2014) Biologically Hazardous Agents at Work and Efforts to Protect Workers' Health: A Review of Recent Reports. Safety and Health at Work 5(2):43–52.
Levy, B. S. and Wegman, D. H. (1994) Occupational Health: Recognizing and Preventing Work-Related Disease. Boston: Little Brown.
Nichols, T. (1998) Health and Safety at Work. Work, Employment & Society 12(2):367–374.
Roh, S. (2012) Work-related diseases of agricultural workers in South Korea. J Korean Med Assoc. 55:1063–1069.
Rosenstock, L. and Cullen, M. R. (1994) Textbook of Clinical Occupational and Environmental Medicine. Philadelphia: Saunders.
Scott, R. M. (2020) Chemical Hazards in the Workplace (e-book). CRC Press.
Spurlock, B. (2017) Physical Hazards of the Workplace. CRC Press.
Wilson, H. G. E. and Agius, R. M. (1994) Health and safety at work. British Medical Journal 309(6948):198–199.

4 Workplace Hazards

Chemical

"There's no better policy in society than pursuing the health and safety of its people"

—Ralph Nader

FACT FILE

- A respirable substance can enter the alveoli and can inhibit with the gas exchange while some respirable substances can enter the bloodstream
- According to WHO an estimated more than 5 million deaths and more than 86 million Disability-Adjusted Life Years (DALYs) are attributable to environmental exposure and management of selected chemicals
- After absorption through skin, chemicals can be transported to body via mucous membranes – the ears, eyes, nose, and mouth
- An inhalable substance can only enter to the extent of bronchioles and get accumulated along the respiratory system and thus affect the mouth, nose, larynx, trachea, and bronchioles
- Chemicals can enter the skin by infiltration, infusion, and assimilation
- Corrosive chemicals can instantly affect living tissue by damaging or destructing the proteins
- Gases can also create long-term or prolonged effects when inhaled or respired, which can have toxic, oncogenic, or mutagenic effects
- Irritants work just like corrosives but produce less acute effects and affect skin and mucous membranes by causing inflammation
- Oils, lubricants, and solvents are common skin irritants which can cause reddening, dryness, and cracking of skin
- The physical state and particle size determine how far chemical substances can enter the respiratory system and beyond
- There are three levels of burns – injury of the epidermis is called a superficial burn and is known as first-degree burn; injury of the dermis is called dermal injury or second-degree burn; and injury of the subcutaneous tissue is known as a full-thickness injury or third-degree burn
- While there are many diverse hazardous workplace chemicals, exposure to these at the workplace can result in various short-term and long-term health effects

DOI: 10.1201/9781003464785-4

4.1 INTRODUCTION

Toxic and hazardous chemicals, mainly as medicines or as poisoning agents, have been of great interest for mankind but seldom as concerns of occupation. In the early 1500s, Swiss physician Philippus Paracelsus recognized that specific chemicals were responsible for the toxicity of poisons and that the human body's reaction to chemicals was dose-dependent. However, it was only in the 19th century that the first structured experimental research was carried out using animals to explore the relationship between chemical exposure and toxic effect. In Germany, Max Gruber published the results of experiments in 1883 on hens and rabbits exposed to carbon monoxide. In the early 1940s, the first list of standards for chemical exposures in industry – Maximum Allowable Concentrations (MACs) was published by the American Conference of Governmental Industrial Hygienists. Hazardous chemicals are among the major hazards that OSH specialists need to deliberate concerning health at the workplace. Hazardous substances are used for a variety of purposes, from simple cleaning to complex chemical processes. Hazardous chemicals may be naturally occurring or man-made, prepared of a single substance or mixture, or can be a by-product of an industrial process. At the workplace, these often produce vapours, fumes, dusts, and mists. A wide range of industrial, laboratory, and farming chemicals, biological agents, and nanoparticles are classified as hazardous which can cause a wide range of health effects, from localized to systemic. While hazardous substances can lead to fire, explosion, and ecological threats, this chapter will only focus on the health risks caused by occupational exposure to hazardous chemicals. Chemicals can exist in many physical states, viz.:

- Solids
- Liquids
- Gases
- Dusts (inhalable and respirable), fumes, vapours, and mists

Depending on environmental factors and/or processes, the physical state of chemicals may change. While assessing the routes of exposure, it is important to consider their characteristics. Substances hazardous to health can be classified as shown in Table 2.1 (Figure 4.1).

Chemical hazards are a major OHS issue around the world. While workers in some industries and some workplaces are at a higher risk of exposure, all workplaces are affected by one or the other type of chemical hazard. Chemical hazards are of two kinds: reactive and toxic. Documenting the toxic effects of chemical hazards need knowledge of acute and chronic exposure and perplexing effect of dormancy in expressing signs and symptoms. While the OHS professionals are likely to address the toxic effects of chemicals, they must be aware of and understand the hazards, risks, and proper control of hazardous chemicals. The classification of chemical hazards is a more methodical approach with the execution of the Globally Harmonised System for Classification and Labelling of Chemicals. Sources of information for identifying hazards include:

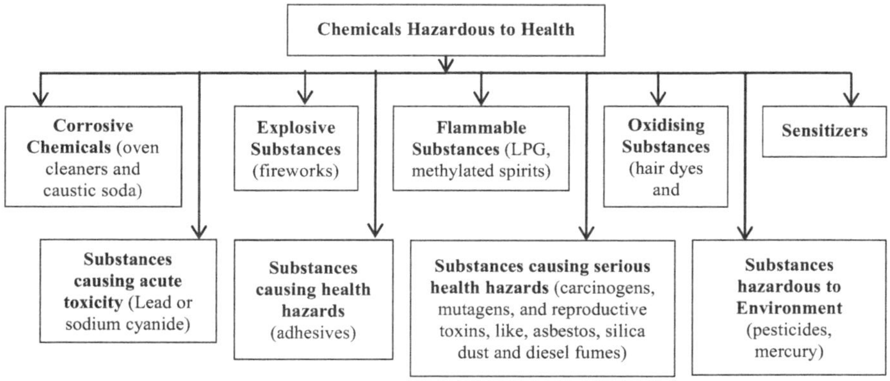

FIGURE 4.1 Classification of substances hazardous to health.

- Chemical label
- Safety data sheet
- Suitable hazardous chemical records

With established exposure standards, these sources offer reference points against which workplace data can be matched. Risk assessment requires knowledge of chemical state, probable routes of absorption, monitoring of exposure, nature of work, and activity undertaken by an employee. Acute toxicity, which refers to "*the adverse health effects after a single or limited number of exposures, can occur after exposure because of equipment failure, insufficient safety during handling or cleaning, or improper management of a chemical*". Though the impact of acute exposures is usually understandable in a short time period, the impact of exposure to some chemicals, such as pesticides, may not appear for several days or months. Temporary effects of acute chemical exposure may include skin irritation, headache, and nausea while lasting effects consist of scars from acid burns. Chronic toxicity refers to "*the adverse health effects after incessant or recurrent exposure over a long time period*", often due to relatively low levels of chemical. There may be a period of dormancy many years before the effects of chronic exposure to a chemical are discovered.

Exposure to Toxic chemicals: One may encounter chemicals such as:

- Reactants
- Solvents
- Catalysts
- Inhibitors
- Starting materials
- Finished products
- By-products
- Contaminants
- Off-specification products

They may vary from pure, single substances to complex branded preparations. Exposures to chemicals may involve:

- Solids
- Liquids
- Airborne matter as mists, aerosols, dusts, fumes (i.e. μm-sized particulates), vapours, or gases in diverse combination

Many circumstances, e.g. exposure to welding fumes or to combustion products of fossil fuels, include combinations both of chemicals and of physical forms. Exposure to a specific chemical in comparatively low concentrations over time may cause chronic effects. At higher concentrations, the effects may be acute. Some chemicals cause local damage at their point of contact or entry in the body; others produce systemic effects, i.e. they circulate in the body and reach various organs before producing an adverse effect. Some airborne chemical contaminants are listed in Table 4.1.

Irritants: Primary irritants cause inflammation, which is one of the body's defence mechanisms. It is basically the reaction of a tissue to harm which is inadequate to kill the tissue and is characterized by:

- Narrowing of small vessels in the affected area
- Dilation of blood vessels
- Increased penetrability of the vessel walls
- Migration of white blood and other defensive cells to the invading harmful chemical

The aim is to concentrate water and protein in the affected area to 'dilute' the effect and wash away the chemical. Production of new cells is accelerated and polluted surface cells are cast off. The respiratory system is the main target organ for vapour, gas, or mist. Promptly-soluble chemicals, e.g. chlorine or phosgene, attack the upper respiratory tract, while the less-soluble gases, e.g. oxides of nitrogen enter more intensely into the airways and may cause pulmonary oedema; e.g. SO_2 is highly water-soluble and is likely to be absorbed in the airways. But, in the presence of particulate chemical agent and sunlight, conversion to SO_3 occurs and the reaction of irritants is more severe. Other body parts are also susceptible:

- the skin and eyes from direct contact/rubbing or from exposure to airborne material including splashes
- the mouth and pharynx by consumption of solid or liquid chemicals

Direct contact of liquid or solid irritants with skin causes contact dermatitis. Some dust can also act as primary irritants. Even chemically inert dusts, e.g. from glass fibres, can induce dermatitis due to abrasion. Examples of primary irritants include acids; alkalis; organic solvents; dehydrating, oxidizing, and reducing agents.

Sensitizers: Generally sensitizers may not produce any ill effects on first contact, though cellular changes can be prompted which may affect the immune system.

TABLE 4.1
Classification of Airborne Contaminants and Their Effects

Classification	Target Organ	Examples
Irritants: Have an eroding or sweltering effect on moist or mucous surfaces.		
(a) Primary	Upper respiratory tract	Chromic acid, Formaldehyde, Gases, Hydrogen chloride, Mists, Sulphur dioxide, Vapour
	Upper and lower respiratory tract	Bromine, Chlorine, Cyanogen chloride, Fluorine, Ozone
	Lower respiratory tract	Arsenic trichloride, Nitrogen dioxide, Phosgene
	Skin	Acids, Alkalis, Chromates, Detergents, Dusts, Inorganic acids (Chromic acid, Nitric acid), Inorganic alkalis (Sodium hydroxide, Sodium carbonate), Organic acids (Acetic acid, Butyric acid), Organic bases (Amines), Organic solvents, Salts (Nickel sulphate, Zinc chloride)
(b) Secondary or allergens	Skin sensitizers	Chlor-2-4-dinitrobenzene, Epoxy-resins Picryl chloride, p-phenyl diamine
	Respiratory sensitizers	Complex salts of platinum, Cyanuric chloride, Isocyanates, p-Phenylene diamine, Proteolytic enzymes
Asphyxiants: Exert an effect by interference with oxidation of tissue. Simple anoxia caused by oxygen deficiency in inhaled air.		
		Aniline, Arsine, Carbon dioxide, Carbon monoxide, Cyanogen, Dimethyl aniline, Helium, Hydrogen, Hydrogen cyanide, Hydrogen sulphide, Methane, Nitrites, Nitrobenzene, Nitrogen, Toluidine
Anaesthetics & Narcotics: Exert effects like simple anaesthesia, by a depressant action on CNS		
		Acetylene, Aliphatic alcohols, Aliphatic ketones, Esters, Ether, Olefins, Paraffin
Systemic Poisons: Cause injury at other than the site of contact.		
	Visceral organs Haematopoietic system Nervous system	Benzene, Carbon disulphide, Halogenated hydrocarbons and metals, Methanol, Organophosphorus compounds, Phenol, Phenols, Tetra-alkyl lead compounds, Toxic inorganic substances, e.g. Pb, Mn, Cd, An, Be, Hg; Ar; P; Se and S compounds and fluorides
Respiratory fibrogens		Asbestos, Fibrogenic dusts, Free crystalline silica, Talc
Carcinogens	Skin	Arsenic, Coal tar pitch dust, Crude anthracene dust, Mineral oil mist
Cancer-causing agents	Respiratory tract	Arsenic, Asbestos, Ether, Mustard gas, Nickel ore, Polycyclic aromatic hydrocarbons
	Liver	Vinyl chloride monomer
	Nasal	Mustard gas, Nickel ore
	Bone marrow	Benzene
Inerts		Argon, Gases, Helium, Hydrogen, Methane, Nitrogen, Particulates

Succeeding exposures to the same, or associated, chemicals may bring about intense allergic reactions. Common industrial skin sensitizers are:

- Coal tar and its direct derivatives
- Dye intermediates
- Dyes
- Explosives
- Insecticides
- Natural resins
- Oils
- Plasticizers
- Synthetic resins

Respiratory sensitizers cause stiffness of chest and seldom a worrying cough but severe cases involve bronchial asthma.

Asphyxiants: Asphyxiants affect the body's oxygen uptake mechanisms. Air usually contains 21 percent oxygen. Oxygen deficiency in inhaled air, e.g. because of the presence of nitrogen, argon, or carbon dioxide in a confined space, depending on the concentration and extent, may affect the body and eventually cause death from simple anoxia.

Anaesthetics and narcotics: Hydrocarbons and certain derivatives, exert a tranquilizing effect on the CNS.

Systemic poisons: These poisons attack organs other than the initial site of contact, including critical organs, viz. kidneys, liver, blood, and bone marrow.

Respiratory fibrogens: This group includes particulate matter which is influenced by the toxicity, size, and morphology of the particle. If dust of specific chemicals is not emptied from the lungs then, over a period, scar tissue may build up, which reduces the elasticity of lungs and impairs breathing. The characteristic disease is classified as pneumoconiosis; common examples are silicosis, asbestosis, coal pneumoconiosis, and talc pneumoconiosis.

Carcinogens: There are certain cancer-causing chemicals, known as carcinogens. Some of the carcinogenic chemicals are listed in Table 4.2.

4.2 TYPES OF CHEMICAL HAZARDS

Any substance, irrespective of its type, that can probably cause a health hazard to individuals, or damage the environment is defined as a chemical hazard. OSHA's Hazard Communication Standard (HCS) defines a hazardous chemical as *'any chemical capable of causing a physical or a health hazard'*. It can also be described as the actual risk linked with specific chemicals, such as:

- Skin blisters
- Long-term undesirable health implications
- Momentary or irreversible ecological damage
- Fire or explosion

TABLE 4.2
Carcinogenic Chemicals

Substance	Site Affected (human)
Chlorambucil, Thiotepa, Cyclophosphamide, Ethylene oxide	Blood
Beryllium and certain compounds	Bone
Acrylonitrile	Colon
Iron dextran	Connective tissue
Ethylene oxide	Gastrointestinal tract
Phenacetin, Cadmium and certain compounds, Auramine, Cyclophosphamide	Kidney, bladder, prostate
Aflatoxins, Carbon tetrachloride, Oxymetholone	Liver
Dimethylcarbamoyl chloride, Dimethyl sulphate, Acrylonitrile, Beryllium and certain compounds, Cadmium and certain compounds	Lung
Nickel and certain compounds	Respiratory tract
Polychlorinated biphenyls	Skin
Amitrole, Polychlorinated biphenyls	Various sites

Types of Chemical Hazards: Although several chemical hazards have been identified and symbolized, the following chemicals are generally found at the workplace:

Explosions and Fires: Explosives are symbolized by an exploding bomb and related to chemicals that may blast or cause mass explosion. Flammable is symbolized with a flame and includes highly flammable gases or chemicals that may catch fire or burn once exposed to air or other explosive sources or elements. Serious fires or explosions are caused by flammable hazardous chemicals. These hazards occur if employees smoke in the area where flammables are stored or in a work operation involving sparks and heat. Mishandling or dropping of large containers can also cause fires and explosions.

Chemical Reactions: On coming in contact with substances, many chemicals react violently; hence, these must be used and stored carefully. Reactions occur after exposure to heat, sunlight, and water or after mixing of certain chemicals.

Environmental Hazards: A symbol of dead tree and fish represents a chemical hazardous to environment. It refers to a chemical that has a lasting damaging effect on the environment. Many chemicals are hazardous to the environment in form of gas and heat emissions; toxin percolation in landfill and waterways; or harm caused by fires, explosions, and chemical reactions which extend outdoor. Many hazards affect human health, plants, wildlife, and microbes, often causing devastation or elimination of entire ecosystems.

Irritants Hazardous to the Ozone Layer: These are usually symbolized by a big exclamation point and refer to chemicals that usually cause inflammation, or rashes in the affected area. These irritants either harm individuals or pose a threat to public health by harming the ozone layer.

Gas under Pressure: It is symbolized by a gas cylinder and pertains to gases which are stored under pressure and may blast when heated or stored at a low temperature causing burns or injury.

Corrosion: It is denoted by corrosion of material and skin and refers to chemicals that can cause skin burns and damage tissue.

Oxidizers: These are represented as a flame over a circle that can cause severe physical hazards such as fires or explosions.

Toxic: It is represented by skull and crossbones, and denotes chemicals that can cause irreversible changes or mutations even at a very low exposure, thereby damaging health, or causing fatality.

Important Hazardous Chemicals: Some of the important hazardous chemicals of concern are listed in Table 4.3:

Other examples of hazardous chemicals at the workplace include gasoline, methanol, disinfectants, glues, cleaning material, detergents, pesticides, paints, cosmetics, welding fumes, metalworking fluids, and heavy metals including lead, aluminium, and mercury.

TABLE 4.3
Important Hazardous Chemicals of Concern

Hazardous Chemicals	Physical State	Workplace Source/Industrial Processes	Health Implications
Ar	Solid	• Farming, wood preservatives • Glass production • Electronics	• Cancer • Damages nervous system • Respiratory and circulatory problems
Benzene	Liquid	• Crude oil and gas • Detergents • Pesticides • Plastics	• Anaemia • Bone marrow damage • Excessive bleeding • Weakened immune system
Cd	Solid	• Rechargeable batteries • Coatings • Solar cells • Pigments • Plastic stabilizers	• Cancer • Damages neurological, reproductive, and gastrointestinal systems • Flu-like symptoms • Kidney and bone disease • Lung and respiratory problems
Cr	Solid	• Industry dealing with coating to prevent rusting of metallic surfaces • Stainless steel industry	• Asthma • Cancer • Damages eyes, eardrums, kidneys, and liver • Respiratory problems
E-Waste	Liquid, solid, gas	Harmful chemicals found in and around disposed appliances such as televisions, fridges, microwaves,	• Cancer • Cardiovascular disease

TABLE 4.3 *(Continued)*
Important Hazardous Chemicals of Concern

Hazardous Chemicals	Physical State	Workplace Source/Industrial Processes	Health Implications
		CPUs, and other household appliances	• Damages DNA, kidney, nervous system • Oxidative stress • Tenderness
Hg	Liquid	• Cosmetics • Dental fillings • Telescopes • Thermometers, barometers, fluorescent lamps, mercury vapour lamp industries • Vaccines	• Harms lungs, thyroid, kidneys, and nervous, digestive and immune systems • Insomnia • Memory loss • Neuromuscular changes • Paralysis • Tremors
Pb	Solid	• Ammunition • Electronics • In-car batteries • Mining sites • Roofing materials • Sailboats • Scuba diving gear	• Anaemia • Birth defects • Brain damage • Kidney disease
Pesticides	Liquid, solid, gas	Agriculture and pesticide production	• Impaired vision • Blisters • Vomiting • Diarrhoea • Respiratory problems • Cancer • Asthma • Seizures • Parkinson's disease
Toluene	Liquid	• Paints, thinners, nail polish removers, inks, stain removers, glues, correction fluids industries • Explosives • Printing works • Leather tanning	• Anxiety • Dermatitis • Giddiness and confusion • Lack of feeling • Liver, and kidney damage • Muscle fatigue • Sleeplessness
Zn	Solid	• Concrete • Ointments • Paints and alloy industries • Pipe organs, auto parts, sensing devices industries • Sunblock	• Cramps • Diarrhoea • Headaches • Kidney and stomach problems • Nausea

4.3 HEALTH AND ECOLOGICAL EFFECTS OF HAZARDOUS CHEMICALS

Release of a hazardous substance can cause health and ecological hazards. Generally, exposure to hazardous chemicals at the workplace can cause adverse health illnesses including headache, difficulty in breathing, skin irritation, severe allergic reaction, and other more serious and long-lasting side effects. There are three ways of exposure to chemicals and pollutants, viz. absorption, ingesting, and inhalation.

Absorption: The workers are exposed to chemicals and pollutants through dermal or eye contact. These organs can be more delicate to chemicals and may react more quickly than the rest of the body.

Ingestion: The workers are exposed to chemicals and pollutants while eating or drinking. Chemicals and pollutants are found in food and water sources.

Inhalation: The workers are exposed to chemicals and pollutants after breathing in. A normal adult breathes 20,000 times a day and this number is much higher for infants and children. The inhaled chemicals and pollutants can end up in the lungs and blood stream. Sometimes, harmful chemicals can be smelled or tasted, but not always, for example, some chemicals like radon or carbon monoxide are odourless, tasteless, and invisible.

General Health Effects: Accidental or incorrect use of workplace chemicals may cause immediate health effects, such as skin or eye irritation or burns, or poisoning. There are long-term health effects of chemicals, which are the result of exposure to workplace chemicals over a long time period. The long-standing health effects include:

- allergies or asthma
- behavioural anomalies
- birth defects
- effect on the mental, intellectual, or physical development of children
- genetic mutations
- malignancy
- organ damage
- physical disabilities
- physiological failures, e.g. kidney failure
- reproductive complications
- weak immune system

4.3.1 Factors Affecting Health Risks of Workplace Chemicals

People respond to chemical exposure in different ways. Some people may come in contact with a chemical but never get harmed, while others may be more sensitive and get sick. Sometimes illness happens only if one is exposed to a harmful substance for a long time. The health risk of chemicals and pollutants depend on several factors, including:

- Duration of contact
- Frequency of exposure

- General well-being of individual
- Mechanism of exposure (through air, products, food, water, and soil)
- Quantity and concentration of the chemical one comes in contact with
- Route of entry
- Type of chemical one is exposed to

Individuals more sensitive to exposure of workplace chemicals and pollutants include:

- Children
- Elderly
- Pregnant people
- Indigenous communities

4.3.2 Health Effects of Workplace Chemicals on Body Systems

The probable health implications of workplace chemicals are discussed according to the body system they affect.

Probable Effects on Respiratory System: Chemical pollutants and their sources affecting the respiratory system are listed in Table 4.4. These result in asbestosis, lung cancer, chronic bronchitis, fibrosis, emphysema, and decreased oxygen supply in blood.

Probable Effects on Excretory System: Chemical pollutants and their sources affecting the excretory system are listed in Table 4.5 and cause decreased formation of urine, decreased blood flow to kidney, decreased ability to filter blood, prevented urine flow, kidney tissue damage, and kidney cancer.

Probable Effects on Cardiovascular System: Chemical pollutants and their sources affecting the cardiovascular system are listed in Table 4.6 and cause heart failure and the inability of blood to carry the necessary oxygen to the body.

Probable Effects on Reproductive System: Chemical pollutants and their sources affecting the reproductive system are listed in Table 4.7 and result in

TABLE 4.4
Chemical Pollutants and Their Sources Affecting Respiratory System

Chemical Pollutants	Sources
Asbestos	Old lining
Benzene	Degreasers
Cd	Old batteries
CO	Car exhaust, faulty furnaces
Ra	Ground
Smoke	Kilns, wood-burning heaters

TABLE 4.5
Chemical Pollutants and Their Sources Affecting Excretory System

Chemical Pollutants	Sources
Cd	Old batteries, cigarette smoke
Chlorinated hydrocarbon solvents	Degreasers, paint removers, dry cleaning solutions
Hg	Thermostats, thermometers, fish living in contaminated water
Pb	Old paint, obsolete plumbing
Ur	Food and water, vicinity to nuclear testing sites

TABLE 4.6
Chemical Pollutants and Their Sources Affecting Cardiovascular System

Chemical Pollutants	Sources
CH_2Cl_2	Auto part cleaners, paint removers
CO	Car exhaust, unvented or faulty furnaces
CS_2	Industrial emissions
Nitrates	Chemical fertilizers

TABLE 4.7
Chemical Pollutants and Their Sources Affecting Reproductive System

Chemical Pollutants	Sources
CH_3Hg	Fish living in polluted water, coal-burning power
CO	Car exhaust, unvented or faulty furnaces
Pb	Old paint, obsolete drainage system

decreased ability to have a baby, increased baby deaths, increased birth defects, and infertility (the inability to have children).

Probable Effects on Nervous System: Chemical pollutants and their sources affecting the nervous system are listed in Table 4.8 and cause loss of feeling, confusion, and decreased speech, sight, memory, muscle strength, or coordination.

Probable Effects on Immune System: Chemical pollutants and their sources affecting the immune system are listed in Table 4.9 and may cause overreaction to environmental substances (allergy), immune system slow down or failure, and autoimmunity (autoimmunity causes the body to attack itself – which makes it more likely to have an over-reaction or infection).

Probable Effects on Skin: Chemical pollutants and their sources affecting the skin are listed in Table 4.10. These can cause irritation, rash, redness, or

TABLE 4.8
Chemical Pollutants and Their Sources Affecting Nervous System

Chemical Pollutants	Sources
Ar	Pressure treated wood
Cd	Discarded batteries
CO	Car exhaust, faulty furnaces
CN	Rat poison

TABLE 4.9
Chemical Pollutants and Their Sources Affecting Immune System

Chemical Pollutants	Sources
Hg	Thermostats, thermometers, some fish
Pb	Old paint, obsolete plumbing
Pesticides	Unwashed fruits and vegetables
Polychlorinated biphenyls (PCBs)	Industrial waste, fish from contaminated water
Polycyclic aromatic hydrocarbons (PAHs)	Cigarette smoke, vehicle exhaust, asphalt roads

TABLE 4.10
Chemical Pollutants and Their Sources Affecting Skin

Chemical Pollutants	Sources
Polychlorinated biphenyls (PCBs)	Industrial waste, fish from contaminated water
Cr	Paints, industrial production
Ar	Pressure treated wood
Hg	Thermostats, thermometers, some fish
Ni	Cement
VOC (Volatile Organic Compounds)	Fumes from gasoline, paint, adhesives, building supplies

discoloration, dermatitis, and health effect related to other systems and organs due to contamination through the skin.

Probable Hepatic Effects: Chemical pollutants and their sources affecting the liver are listed in Table 4.11 and cause liver damage, tumours, accumulation of fat, and death of liver cells.

Likewise, the impacts of chemical emissions released from industrial units and agriculture farms on the environment can be distressing, affecting aquatic life, damaging animals and plants in a polluted area, causing major reproductive problems in animals, or else limit the capacity of an ecosystem to endure. Some

TABLE 4.11
Chemical Pollutants and Their Sources Affecting Liver

Chemical Pollutants	Sources
CCl_4	Adhesives
CH_2Cl_2	Auto part cleaners, paint removers
C_2H_3Cl	Pipe sealer

hazardous chemicals also have the potential to blow up or cause a fire, intimidating both animal and human populations.

4.3.3 Chemical Risk Assessment

Chemical risk assessment involves knowledge of how much a particular chemical can cause a hazard and whether there is likelihood of exposure to that chemical to exceed the permissible level. Where there is evidence of workers' exposure to a hazardous chemical or release of such a chemical into the atmosphere and the controls are known, the OHS professional may go monitor the exposure. But, there are circumstances when this simplistic approach is not suitable. Chemical risk assessment is more than allocating a rating. The risk of harm or damage from chemical exposure is multifactorial, and is a function of the:

- chemical state
- dose-response relationship
- extent of exposure
- individual worker
- nature of task or activity involving the chemical
- route of exposure
- workplace environment

The sources of information for hazard identification discussed above also give input for risk assessment. However, attentiveness, vigilance, and supporting information are vital while relating the data of such sources for chemical risk assessment.

Chemical State: While chemical hazard identification is about identifying the chemical as a probable source of harm, evaluating the risk involves knowledge of how the chemical acts and how it might cause harm. The state (e.g. solid, liquid, or gas) in which the chemical is used is one cause that can affect the level of risk, for example, in case of most dust, the finer the dust, the more toxic and irritable it is, and the more likely it stays in air and enter the lungs.

Routes of Exposure: For many chemicals, the risk level depends on the route of exposure. Hazardous chemicals can enter the body through the respiratory tract, via inhalation, dermal contact, and the digestive tract, via ingestion, or via injection directly into the bloodstream. Usually, inhalation is the most important route of exposure for chemical risk assessment. However, some chemicals, e.g. pesticides, can be absorbed through skin. Chemicals can be ingested while consuming food or smoking with contaminated hands. Thus, though exposure standards tend to focus on inhalation exposure, the OHS expert needs to be aware of other potential exposure routes.

Dose-response: It is the amount of the material likely to produce an effect, and is an important component of chemical risk assessment. Increasing doses of toxic chemicals cause increased seriousness of health implications. Use of the globally harmonized system (GHS) efficiently eliminates the necessity to consider the dose-response relationship as part of chemical risk assessment.

Level of Exposure: Concentration, rate of recurrence, and length of exposure affect the risk of damage. Exposure to a chemical may be evaluated in one or more of three ways:

1. Inspection and observation provide information on the risk associated with use of chemicals and involves:
   - Formal workplace inspections
   - Observation of work tasks
   - *'Walk-through'* inspections

   Visible pollution, spills, and storage issues specify the likelihood of inhalation, skin contact, or hazardous interactions, e.g. contact between flammable materials and sources of ignition. Inspections and maintenance records provide important information on capability of controls, such as ventilation, for instance, odour may indicate the presence of a chemical in the air; however, some chemicals have poor warning properties, in that they are toxic before the odour is perceptible, e.g. carbon monoxide.
2. Incident and first aid reports, viz. reports of incidents, e.g. fires or spills and complaints of health effects, e.g. skin irritation or respiration problems provide information required for chemical hazard identification.
3. While there is evidence of worker exposure to or release of toxic chemicals into the atmosphere, the OHS expert may follow the instant control and monitoring of exposure, or may regulate and control the extent of exposure using monitoring equipment. There are numerous simple devices for assessing ambient air contamination. Monitoring involves an understanding of sampling requirements to address all probable exposure impacts throughout the '*lifecycle*' of the task, including maintenance and cleaning.

Task or activity: Aspects of a work task may affect the level of exposure and consequently the risk, for example, farmers are at higher risk of chemical exposure linked with the use of pesticides. Exposure to two or more chemicals produces the probability for them to react '*synergistically*;' i.e. the health impacts of two chemicals together are greater than that of the individual chemicals alone, for example, carbon tetrachloride and ethanol are separately toxic to the liver, but together they cause more liver injury than the sum of their individual effects.

Workplace Environment: A variety of factors at the workplace may impact exposure to a chemical. These factors may vary seasonally, and depend on maintenance periods or other activities in the area, and may include:

- Environmental circumstances, viz. temperature, sunlight, and humidity
- Potential contact with adjacent processes or incompatible chemicals
- Sources of explosion

Worker: Workers' exposure to a chemical depends on their:

- role in the task or activity
- training and skills
- use of personal protective equipment (PPE)

Also, individual vulnerability is governed by factors, such as:

- Alcohol consumption
- General health status
- Genetic factors
- Pregnancy
- Smoking
- Use of medications and drugs

An individual's status in terms of these aspects may not be easily understandable, but may be detected by an occupational health practitioner.

Risk Communication: Communication with employees, administrators, and directors about chemical hazards, probable and real exposures, and the need for monitoring is vital. Exposure monitoring data must be shared with those probably exposed and those involved in the assessment. While communicating information about the risk of chemical hazards, the reason of ambient monitoring and biological monitoring, the inadequacies and ambiguities linked with the information, and effects of exposure must be defined.

4.4 REGULATING EXPOSURE TO CHEMICAL HAZARDS AT WORKPLACE

Workstations and factories, mainly the manufacturing or other related industries – can't eliminate completely or avoid the use of hazardous chemicals. However, they can follow and observe safety measures aimed at regulating chemical hazards at the workplace and reduce their potential harmful impact on workers. Of all preventive measures to pro-actively maintaining a safe working environment, identification of hazardous chemicals at the workplace is the most important. Some of these are evident and easy to identify, while others are not evident. Once the potential hazards are recognized, there must be an assessment of the risks linked with the chemicals, together with likelihood of occurrence of risks. The next step involves management or control of identified risks. While dealing with chemical hazards at the workplace, the following principle of the hierarchy of control must be followed:

Elimination: Totally remove and suspend the use of the hazardous chemicals

Substitution: Finding substitutes or replace with other less hazardous chemicals

Engineering Control: Execute changes in the process, for example, decreasing contact with the chemicals, or physically detaching people from them

Administrative Control: Execute changes in the way people work, such as rotation of schedules or reorganizing job assignments

Personal Protective Equipment (PPE): In case the hazardous chemicals can't be avoided, or the contact of employees can't be reduced, the use of PPE can be ensured to lessen the exposure and risk factors. The best way to control chemical hazards at the workplace is to develop a consistent chemical management procedure

The four important steps to Chemical Management Procedure are:

Step 1: Classification: Classifying each workplace chemical, to get an understanding of both health and physio-chemical hazards.

Step 2: Evaluation: Conducting a risk evaluation of each hazardous chemical, taking into account the probability of accidents or hazardous events that could occur along with possible consequences.

Step 3: Control: Using the hierarchy of controls, introduce changes in the workplace to eliminate or minimize exposure to the hazard.

Step 4: Sustain: Having an equipped system to assess the control measures and classify, evaluate, and regulate any new chemicals that are introduced to the workplace.

Safe Storage of Hazardous Chemicals: It involves a special plan for safe storage of chemicals. An essential part of a Chemical Management Plan is checking that the workplace has safe chemical storage area and safety cabinets suitable for each chemical substance. This could include:

- Acid storage cabinets
- Corrosive cupboards
- Gas bottle crates
- Hazardous goods containers
- Inflammable cabinets
- Pesticide storage cupboards
- PPE cabinets

These cabinets must be kept in well-ventilated areas either inside or outside. Aeration is a main factor for storage of hazardous chemicals and risk assessment defines whether chemical stores are positioned indoor or outdoor. Chemical safety cabinets are suggested for they are built from well-suited material displaying all mandatory posters, labels, and signage. Industries must have all-inclusive and standard control measures that can be obeyed by involving workers and organizations to avoid any hazardous results of chemicals. Implementing and continuing the right control measures include constant training and review. Safety audits can be a decisive factor to know which control measures work and which don't.

Assessment of Efficiency of Control: Once executed, the efficiency of controls must be assessed. Data on efficacy of controls may be gathered in a number of ways:

- Biological monitoring of urine, blood, exhaled breath, hair, or saliva samples from possibly exposed individuals
- Medical investigation, together with monitoring the exposed population for genuine health effects due to exposure
- Regular ambient air quality monitoring to assess whether air concentrations are retained below the suggested limits
- Reporting and investigation of falls, leaks, damages of control, environmental releases, or OESs being exceeded
- Walk-through surveys to spot the correct handling of material and use of engineering, administrative, and PPE controls

Undertaking and inferring the outcomes of assessment activities call for an occupational hygiene specialist and knowledge of occupational health.

BIBLIOGRAPHY

Allen, D. T. and Rosselot, K. S. (1996) Pollution Prevention for Chemical Processes. New York: Wiley.

Armour, M. A. (1996) Hazardous Laboratory Chemicals Disposal Guide. CRC Press: Lewis Publishers.

Bayley, J. (1991) Health and safety at work. British Dental Journal 170(10):364–365.

Boleij, J. S. M. *et al.* (1994) Occupational Hygiene of Chemical and Biological Agents. Amsterdam: Elsevier Science Ltd.

Borzelleca, J. F. (1999) Paracelsus: Herald of modern toxicology. Toxicological Sciences 53(1):2–4.

Bourdeau, P. and Green, G. (1989) Methods for Assessing and Reducing Injury from Chemical Accidents. Chichester: Wiley.

Bretherick, L. (1990) Handbook of Reactive Chemical Hazards. Oxford: Butterworth-Heinemann.

Carson, P. and Mumford, C. (2002) Hazardous Chemicals Handbook. Oxford: Butterworth-Heinemann.

Carson, P. A. and Mumford, C. J. (1996) The Safe Handling of Chemicals in Industry. Harlow: Longman Scientific and Technical.

Cheremisinoff, P. N. and Graffia, M. (1995) Safety Management Practices for Hazardous Materials. New York: Marcel Dekker.

Collins, L. R. and Schneid, T. D. (2001) Physical hazards of the workplace. Boca Raton, FL: Lewis Publishers.

Crowl, D. A. and Louvar, J. F. (2011) Chemical Process Safety: Fundamentals with Applications. Boston, MA: Prentice Hall.

Cutler, R. (1991) Health and safety at work. British Dental Journal 170(7):251.

Fraser, T. M. (1996) Toxic Chemicals in the Workplace. Houston, TX: Gulf Publishing.

Grandjean, P. (1990) Skin Penetration, Hazardous Chemicals at Work. London: Taylor and Francis.
Greenberg, M. I. (1997) Occupational, Industrial and Environmental Toxicology. St Louis: Mosby.
Hernberg, S. (1992) Introduction to Occupational Epidemiology. Philadelphia: Lewis Publishers.
Hopkins, A. (2005) Safety, Culture and Risk: The Organisational Causes of Disasters. Sydney, NSW: CCH Australia.
King, R. W. and Magid, J. (1979) Industrial Hazard and Safety Handbook. London: Newnes-Butterworth.
Levy, B. S. and Wegman, D. H. (1994) Occupational Health: Recognizing and Preventing Work-Related Disease. Boston: Little Brown.
Lewis, P. (1993) Health Protection from Chemicals in the Workplace. Chichester: Ellis Horwood Ltd.
Nichols, T. (1998) Health and safety at work. Work, Employment & Society 12(2):367–374.
Robinson, L. and Thorn, I. (2005) Toxicology and Ecotoxicology in Chemical Safety Assessment. Oxford, UK: Blackwell Publishing.
Rosenstock, L. and Cullen, M. R. (1994) Textbook of Clinical Occupational and Environmental Medicine. Philadelphia: Saunders.
Scott, R. M. (2020) Chemical Hazards in the Workplace (e-book). Boca Raton: CRC Press.
Snedeker, S. M. (2006) Chemical exposures in the workplace: Effect on breast cancer risk among women. American Association of Occupational Health Nurses Journal 54(6):270–279.
Spurlock, B. (2017) Physical Hazards of the Workplace. Boca Raton: CRC Press.
Thoreau, H. D. (1981) Occupational health risks and the worker's right to know. Yale Law Journal 90(8):1792–1810.
Tillman, C. (2007) Principles of Occupational Health and Hygiene: An Introduction. Crows Nest, NSW: Allen & Unwin.
Wilson, H. G. E. and Agius, R. M. (1994) Health and safety at work. BMJ 309(6948):198–199.

5 Workplace Hazards

Physical and Ergonomic

"A positive working environment is a workplace that promotes employee safety, growth, and goal attainment. stimulating"

—Anonymous

FACT FILE

- Noise exposure above 85 dB (A) may cause short-term or permanent hearing damage
- Noises of frequencies above 1–2 kHz are found to be unsafe and increase the risk of hearing loss
- Shots of a high sound pressure level above 160 dB can cause permanent hearing impairment
- Tinnitus occurs when the frequency of sound is above 1 kHz
- Physiological disorders may arise when the sound level exceeds 75 dB
- Strong acoustic stimuli above 110–120 dB may impact the functioning vision, balance, or tactile sensation
- Weaker acoustic stimuli of 55–75 dB may result in the loss of concentration, making performance of work difficult and decreasing efficiency
- For every doubling of the distance between the noise source and employee, the noise level is reduced by 6 dBA
- Ionizing radiation is a type of ray released by atoms in the form of electromagnetic waves
- Low doses of ionizing radiation increase the risk of long-term effects, for instance, cancer
- Heat stress can arise from pronged work in full personal protective equipment
- Working outdoors in extreme cold or heat can cause serious health damage
- Poor lighting at the workplace can cause injuries, eye strain, and loss of vision

5.1 INTRODUCTION

Workplace hazards occur when the working setting can cause injury, disease, or death. These hazards can be the resultant of different facets of the working environment, including equipment, hazardous materials, risky working practices,

DOI: 10.1201/9781003464785-5

and the conduct of people. Workplace hazards are also a common cause of physical injuries. A hazard that can cause physical harm to an employee is known as physical hazard and can be found both in natural and workplace environment, including construction sites, workshops, and offices. It is important to recognize workplace physical hazards so as to control or eliminate them. Likewise, an ergonomic hazard denotes any physical condition or factor at the workplace that can cause short and long-term injury or health implications.

To begin with, most ergonomic hazards affect the musculoskeletal system, producing aches or strains that may seem to be small and irrelevant, but with passage of time can become serious ailments that can cause permanent damage to the body. It is important to seriously consider the workplace ergonomic hazards because a small muscle strain can ultimately become a long-term health problem. If these workplace hazards are left unattended, they can cause injuries and illnesses that have implications on workers both at the physical and mental levels. This chapter discusses important physical and ergonomic hazards.

5.2 DUST AS WORKPLACE HAZARD

Dust is one of the most injurious agents present in the work environment. Dust is a general term that refers to solid particles of varying size and origin, which remain suspended in a gas for a period of time; while particle is a small, separate part of a solid or liquid substance and nanoparticle is a nano-object with three-dimensions in the nano-scale. Human exposure to dust can cause mechanical injury of the mucosa or skin, allergic reactions and diseases, pneumoconiosis, and cancer. Industrial units emit harmful dusts in the working environment but their concentration and harmful impacts on human health depend on work processes. Though the concentration of dust in offices is much lower than in industrial setups, the concentration, particle size, and distribution of dust are still important in the context of '*sick building syndrome*'. Recent studies on the harmful effects of dust containing minute particles, viz. particles with nano-metric dimensions, show them to have serious health implications. These particles are released in the processes of welding, soldering, burning of motor oils, and smoking. Nowadays, the focus is on the harmful effects of nanoparticles that are emitted during the nano-technological processes. Nanoparticles are known to induce an inflammatory reaction in the alveoli and cause blood clotting. These particles enter the human body mainly through the respiratory system, but they can also be found in the liver.

Sources: Depending on the source of emission, dust emitted at workstations can have different properties. Sources of dust emission at the workplace include the following:

- Technological processes
- Personnel handling machines and equipment
- Air supplied from the outside by forced air ventilation unit or by infiltration
- Nano-technological processes

Based on the following parameters, the degree of human exposure can be assessed:

- Chemical configuration and crystal structure (e.g. crystalline silica or amorphous silica)
- Concentration of dust (concentration of dust particles of different sizes)
- Explosive properties of the dust (e.g. wood dust or flour dust)
- Particle shape (fibrous and non-fibrous dusts)
- Particle size (coarse-, medium-, and fine-dispersed dust)

Assessment of Occupational Risk Linked with Dust: The assessment of occupational risk related with dust exposure is a complex process. Estimation of dust exposure is done through:

- Grouping the category of dust present at the workplace
- Assessment of the chemical composition and concentration of dust
- Estimation of the dust exposure index
- Comparison of the obtained exposure index values with the permissible concentration values
- Valuation of the occupational risk linked with dust exposure
- Measurement of risk permissibility

Risk Reduction: It is one of the most important means to ensure occupational safety and health. Employees' protection against the detrimental effects of dust requires the following:

- Application of collective protection against dust
- Assessing the occupational risks of workers exposed to harmful dust
- Determining the category, concentration, and other basic parameters of dust
- Estimating employees' exposure to harmful dust
- Eliminating or regulating the dust exposure of employees
- Use of appropriate personal protection equipment

Collective Protection against Dust: This includes:

- Devices well-equipped with air filters
- General and Local mechanical ventilation systems

The purpose of ventilation systems is as follows:

- To improve the condition and composition of air at workstations according to identified needs for safety of human health and the technology required for production of products with specific properties.
- To normalize air parameters, including pollution concentration, temperature, humidity, velocity, and direction of movement of air.

5.3 VIBROACOUSTIC HAZARDS

Vibroacoustics is a discipline of science that deals with vibration and acoustic processes observed in life and workplace environment including nature, engineering machines and equipment, means of transportation, and communication. Exposure to noise and vibration at the workplace can cause Vibroacoustic hazards. From the perspective of occupational and health safety, vibration is a set of phenomena observed at workstations, generating the transmission of energy from the source of vibration to the human body through various body parts that come in contact with the oscillating source while completing the tasks. Permanent occupational exposure to vibration may lead to many disorders and cause permanent pathological changes. The type of changes and the pace of their development depend on the point of permeation to the human body. In this regard, two types of mechanical vibration can be distinguished:

Whole-Body Vibration: Affects the human body in general, entering through the legs, pelvis, back, or the sides

Hand-Arm Vibration: Acts on the human body through the upper limbs.

To assess the impact of mechanical vibration on the human body, vibration acceleration is generally measured for it provides the best characterization of the energy-related aspects of the vibration process. This quantity is linked with the accepted permissible values relating to daily exposure of 8 hours.

Impacts of Vibroacoustic Hazards on Human Body: Mechanical vibration passed on from oscillatory systems to the human body may have a negative impact on individual systems and organs, or it may cause whole body vibration or its parts and cellular structures. Long-standing exposure to vibration may lead to many disorders and cause perpetual and irreversible pathological changes. However, these changes depend on the type of vibration to which an individual is exposed – whole-body or hand-arm vibration.

Hand-Arm Vibration: Exposure to vibration transmitted to the organism through the upper limbs – hand-arm vibration causes pathological changes in:

- Circulatory system
- Nervous system
- Osteo-articular system

Epidemiological research has shown a relationship between pathological changes and work conditions. Thus, a set of these changes, known as vibration syndrome, is considered an occupational disease. The vascular form of vibration syndrome is the most frequent and is categorized by changes mostly in peripheral blood circulation in the form of paroxysmal vaso-spastic disorders of upper extremities (white fingers). Paroxysmal vasospasms are indicated by one or more fingertips turning pale. This vibration syndrome is often confused with Raynaud's disease.

Vaso-spastic disorders are often supplemented by nervous disorders and osteo-articular changes. Changes in the nervous system caused by exposure to hand-arm vibration mostly include pallesthesia, apselaphesia, loss of sense of temperature, and related problems such as numbness or tingling of fingertips. If exposure continues, these changes develop further, diminishing the ability to work and perform other life functions. Operators of manual vibration tools are the main group exposed to hand-arm vibration. Osteo-articular changes in the hand are caused mainly by hand-arm vibration of frequency below 30 Hz, including:

- Calcification of articular capsules
- Changes in the periosteum and woven bone
- Development of characteristic cysts in small bones, mainly in the wrist
- Malformation of articular spaces

Whole-Body Vibration: The negative effects of occupational exposure to whole-body vibration are mostly related to:

- Skeletal system
- Internal organs

In the skeletal system, pathological changes develop mostly in the lumbar segment of spine, and less often in the cervical segment. Spinal pain syndrome because of pathological changes in people occupationally exposed to whole body vibration has been recognized as an occupational disease – like vibration syndrome caused by hand-arm vibration. Internal organ disorders caused by whole-body vibration are mostly because of the resonance excitation of individual organs. This produces harmful changes in the functioning of the alimentary system organs, mainly the stomach and the oesophagus, besides organs of the thorax, female reproductive system, and nasopharyngeal cavity. Construction and road machine operators and car, tram, and engine drivers are exposed to whole-body vibration. In this case, vibration is transferred to the body from the vehicle seat through the pelvis, back, and sides. Occupational exposure to whole-body vibration often affects persons who operate fixed equipment and machines in a standing position. In such a case, vibrations enter an employee's body through the feet from the vibrating base of the workstation. The effect of these vibrations is similar to those conveyed by seats. The biological effects of hand-arm and whole-body vibrations on the human body are generally supplemented by functional effects, which include the following:

- Annoyance
- Extreme lethargy
- Insomnia
- Movement coordination disorders
- Prolonged motor and visual response time

Undesirable functional changes decrease the efficiency and quality of the work performance, occasionally making it difficult to work at all. Since mechanical vibration and its effects are common in the work environment, it must be assessed to evaluate the occupational risk and to lessen the risk level. Data regarding the emission of vibration from machine is important for engineers, builders, workers, and scrutiny specialists, and is essential for comparing the vibration emitted by various machines and for the estimation of vibrations to conform to the needs of occupational health and safety.

Sources of Vibrations: Vibration sources in the workplace environment can be divided into two groups:

Whole-Body Vibration Sources

- Floors and podiums in buildings and other amenities on which the work-stations are positioned; the main sources of vibration in this case are mobile, portable, or fixed devices and machines, operated inside or outside, which cause vibration of the floor on which the operator is standing
- Oscillating podiums
- Seats and floors of construction
- Seats and floors of transport vehicles

Hand-Arm Vibration Sources

- Inflated, hydraulic, or electric hand-held impact tools (moulding hammers, riveting hammers, hammer drills, wrenches)
- Electric- or diesel-powered hand-held rotary tools (drills, grinders, chainsaws)
- Hand-operated control levers of machines and vehicles
- Technological process sources (hand-held or hand-guided components processed by grinding, smoothing, polishing, etc.)

Some hand-operated tools, such as hammers and mechanical saws, can create high vibration acceleration, which may be transferred through shoulders to torso and head, causing resonance excitation in the internal organs. Therefore, hand-held tools are whole body vibration sources.

Preventive Measures: Methods of avoiding, reducing, and restraining vibration exposure can be divided into technical and organizational methods. The technical methods include:

- Active control of vibration
- Limiting vibration along its propagation route
- Mechanization of technological processes using remote control of vibration sources
- Removal or restriction of vibration at the source

The vibro-activity of the sources may be reduced by:

- Automation of technological processes and remote control of vibration sources let the workers be away from the areas exposed to mechanical vibration
- Changing the structure, proper assembly, or fixing the machines to the floor
- Employing expansion joints separating the foundations of machines and devices from the surrounding area
- Using personal protection equipment, such as anti-vibration gloves
- Using vibro-isolation materials (mats, washers, special vibration isolators)

The vibro-activity of sources can be diminished by:

- Altering the internal structure of the vibration source
- Changing the parameters of the vibration exciting force
- Decreasing clearances to a minimum
- Eliminating micro-impacts
- Fixing the machine to the floor
- Refining balancing, and removing mutual impact of cooperating components

5.4 NOISE AS WORKPLACE HAZARD

Noise is defined as an undesirable, unkind, annoying, trying, or injurious sound that touches the hearing organ and affects other senses and organs of the human body. In physical terms, sound is a mechanical vibration of an elastic medium (gas, liquid, or solid). The vibration may be regarded an oscillatory movement of particles in a medium with respect to the equilibrium condition, causing a change in the atmospheric pressure. The variation of pressure or disturbance from equilibrium is transferred as a resultant local condensation and rarefaction of the medium's particles in the space adjacent to the vibrating source, creating an acoustic wave. Based on the frequency range, noise is classified as follows:

- Audible noise (with a spectrum of audible frequencies between 16 and 16,000 Hz)
- Infrasonic noise (with a spectrum of infrasound frequencies between 1 and 20 Hz)
- Ultrasonic noise (with a spectrum of high audible frequencies and low ultrasound frequencies, between 10 and 40 kHz)

Noise can be classified on the basis of causes or sources, viz. aerodynamic noise: produced by a flow of air or other gases, and mechanical noise, produced as a result of friction and impacts of machine parts. Noise can also be categorized by the environment in which it is perceived; for example, noise in an industrial environment is known as industrial noise, noise in residential areas/public spaces/ recreational areas is known as community noise, and noise produced due to transport is known as transport noise.

Sources of Noise: The three most harmful sources of noise pollution in an industrial setting are machinery, construction, and vehicles. People working with drills, punch presses, saws, mills, etc. are exposed to noise pollution. Mechanical pneumatic drills, saws, and rotating belts can create unbearably high levels of sound that can annoy the public and harmfully affect the employees of engineering companies, textile mills, and metalworking factories. Likewise, workers involved in construction, blasting, demolishing, mining, and other similar activities are exposed to high intensity of noise pollution. There are many sources of noise, but some of them are:

Traffic Noise: Traffic noise accounts for most polluting noise in cities and traffic police and workers working on the roadside are exposed to traffic noise.

Air Traffic Noise: Though there are fewer aircraft that fly over towns than there are cars on the roads, the impact is greater.

Construction Sites: Workers involved in building, park construction, road, and pavement resurfacing works are exposed to noisy environment.

Besides this, bars, restaurants, and terraces including pubs and clubs that spill outside produce noise that affects the employees working in the pubs and clubs and surrounding areas are exposed to noisy music. Noise made by animals can go unnoticed, but a howling or barking dog, for example, can produce around 60–80 dB.

Health Implications of Noise: The adverse effects of noise on human beings are linked mostly with the hearing organ, but non-auditory effects are observed in the entire body. Short-term exposure to loud noise can also cause a temporary change in hearing or cause tinnitus. The short-term complications may go away within a few minutes or hours after leaving the noise source; yet, recurrent exposure to loud noise can lead to permanent tinnitus and/or hearing loss. Loud noise, by making it difficult to catch the warning signals, can:

- Add to workplace accidents and injuries
- Decrease efficiency
- Inhibit communication and concentration
- Induce physical and psychological stress

The impact of noise-induced hearing loss can be intense, restricting one's capacity to hear high-frequency sounds, and understand speech, and seriously impairing one's capacity to talk. Noise health effects can be the physical and psychological health consequences of constant exposure to elevated sound levels. According to the World Health Organization, after air pollution, noise from traffic is one of the worst environmental stressors for humans. Raised workplace or environmental noise can cause:

- Annoyance
- Birth defects
- Changes in the immune system
- Vasoconstriction and cardiovascular effects
- Hearing impairment
- Hypertension
- Ischaemic heart disease
- Sleep disturbance
- Tinnitus

Although age-related health effects are obvious with progressing age, in many nations the collective impact of noise is enough to cause hearing impairment in a large section of population over the years. Chronic exposure to noise is linked with insomnia and increased incidence of diabetes. By reason of chronic exposure to noise the sympathetic nervous system's inability to acclimatize results in adverse cardiovascular effects. The sympathetic nervous system retains lighter stages of sleep but when the body is exposed to noise, the blood pressure rises and falls affecting the circadian rhythm.

Effect of Noise on Auditory Organs: When the hearing organ is exposed to excessive noise, the hearing threshold is raised, which may be rescindable, a momentary threshold shift, or permanent, after many years of hazardous exposure, and may occur in diverse frequencies. In both cases, the indicator is difficulty in hearing. A temporary threshold shift reduces after the noise ceases; a permanent threshold shift is irreparable and does not show any retrieval over time. A temporary threshold shift starts after long exposure to noise at more than 75–80 dB and increases rapidly with an increased noise level. The increase is in both the size of temporary threshold move in decibels and the recovery time must be restored for normal hearing. Temporary threshold shift is regarded as a temporary loss of hearing. It may occur because of hearing fatigue after long exposure to noise or because of an acute acoustic trauma caused by a sudden or impulsive noise. A temporary threshold shift is the first indication that the adjacent noise may pose a threat to hearing. A permanent threshold shift is an irreparable damage to the hearing organ. The risk of long-lasting hearing damage starts when the sound level exceeds 80–85 dB. Feebler stimuli do not harm the auditory organ even after long and constant exposure.

Hearing damage is generally an outcome of long-term exposure to noise, as the result on the hearing organ is added over the time. Auditory loss is linked to the amount of acoustic energy received by the hearing organ in a certain time period. Furthermore, constant exposure to noise is more damaging than intermittent exposure, for hearing regeneration can start even during short breaks. Increase in the hearing threshold is analysed using audiometric tests, which can detect hearing threshold changes of only several decibels that may not be perceived by the patient. Small changes do not remarkably impair hearing ability. These changes are typical in the early period of noise-induced hearing damagė, which progresses gradually and constantly. Audiometric tests also show the development of permanent hearing loss. To a great extent, the type of hearing loss depends on its cause. In chronic noise exposure, hearing loss often starts in a high frequency range (4–6 kHz) and then continues to lower frequencies. Medium- and high-frequency noise is considered more unsafe than noise with a low-frequency maximum energy. This is because of the frequency-dependent sensitivity of the ear, which is the maximum in the frequency range of 3–5 kHz. Individual vulnerability to noise varies depending on the genetic factors and previous incidence of disease. Hearing damage may also be due to sudden damage to the hearing organ causing acoustic trauma or acute acoustic trauma. A sudden noise in a broad frequency range produces acoustic trauma, and an abrupt increase in the noise level to above 130–140 dB can result in acute acoustic trauma. Noises of frequencies above 1–2 kHz are found to be unsafe and increase the risk of hearing loss. These frequencies are caused by electronic sound generation devices. Acoustic trauma is often caused by shots and explosions. In spite of short-term exposure, shots of a high sound pressure level above 160 dB can cause permanent hearing impairment. Noise causes irreversible damage mostly to the hair cells of the inner ear. In extreme cases, a blast resulting in a shock wave of a peak sound pressure level exceeding 180 dB may cause defects and puncturing of the tympanic membrane and can harm the auditory ossicles in the middle ear.

Hearing loss is not the only result of noise. Exposure to noise may also result in a substantial increase in the frequency and intensity of tinnitus. Tinnitus is the occurrence of whistling and buzzing sounds, generally of a frequency above 1 kHz, which are not present physically but are personally heard and are generated at various levels of the hearing system. Exposure to extreme noise can cause hypersensitivity to sound and the person finds it problematic to bear sounds and perceives them as annoying even if they are soft by normal standards. Permanent cochlear hearing loss results in a loss of the ability to understand speech and is a lasting infirmity for which there is no therapy. This has long surpassed the listing of work-related diseases.

Non-auditory Impacts of Noise: Non-auditory effects of noise are not yet documented completely. The structural link between the hearing nerve tract and the cortex permits hearing stimuli to influence other centres of the brain and endocrine system and, consequently, the condition and functioning of many internal organs. Sound stimuli may thus affect the functioning of the body of an organism. This has been established by reflexive actions of the respiratory, circulatory, and digestive systems, and many other organs in response to noise. Instances of non-auditory physiological responses include:

- Change in body posture after an unforeseen explosion
- Contraction of peripheral blood vessels
- Motor reflexes after an unpredicted explosion

- Muscle contractions after an unexpected explosion
- Reduced intensity of intestinal peristalsis
- Reduced rate of respiration

Preventive Measures: Non-auditory noise effects are a general response to noise as a stressor. These values are relevant in all types of noise, viz. stable, unstable, and impulse. High-tech means of inhibiting, removing, or regulating noise exposure are based on the instantaneous application of mechanical, organizational, and administrative resolutions, which are based on a detailed analysis of the acoustic conditions at workplaces with extreme noise. There are several methods to regulate and decrease exposure to noise in a workstation, for instance:

Engineering controls involve amending or substituting equipment, or making linked physical changes at the noise source or along the transmission route to lessen the noise level at the employee's ear. The operational engineering controls include:

- Enfold or segregate noise source by keeping a barricade between source of noise and worker
- Maintain and grease machinery and equipment
- Select low-noise apparatus and machinery

Administrative controls are modifications in the workstation or schedule that lessen or remove the employee's exposure to noise. The administrative controls include:

- Offer silent zones where employees can get a break from risky noise source;
- Regulating noise exposure through distance is often an operational, yet simple and cost-effective administrative mechanism;
- Restricting the time duration a person is exposed to a noise source; and
- Running noisy machines in shifts to lessen the exposure

5.5 ELECTROMAGNETIC FIELDS AS WORKPLACE HAZARD

Since antiquity, electromagnetic fields (EMFs) are present in nature. Geo-static magnetic fields, the electric fields of Earth's atmosphere, and low-frequency magnetic fields exist in the natural environment. According to the U.S. National Institute for Occupational Safety and Health, every person is exposed to EMFs due to the presence of electric devices around each one of us. The incidence of exposure to electric fields and low frequency magnetic fields at workstations can reach nearly 100 percent of workers in cities. The properties of EMF are generally evaluated with reference to its two components, viz. electric field and magnetic field. The magnetic field is present around moving electric charges or because of the magnetisation of some material. The electric field occurs both around moving and stationary charges. The exposure level is generally defined by:

- Electric field strength (E)
- Frequency (f)
- Magnetic field strength (H)

These fields are present in the workplace which affects the employee's body. The intensity of electromagnetic hazard is governed by the polarisation and spatial distribution of the field with regard to the human body and the link between the strengths of the electric and magnetic fields. The energy of electric fields has an impact both on moving and stationary charges, while the magnetic fields only disturb moving charges.

Sources of EMFs: EMFs are unnoticed lines of force created when electricity is produced or used. EMFs are produced by:

- Dielectric heaters for joining plastic elements
- Drills, copy machines, electric pencil sharpeners
- Electrical equipment and appliances like electrical wiring
- Electrical appliances including office or computer equipment
- Electrochemical devices, for instance electrolytic vats
- Electro-thermal devices, such as arc furnaces and induction furnaces
- Heaters for thermal processing of steel elements
- Induction heaters
- Industrial magnetisers and demagnetisers
- Large electric motors and generators
- Lighting equipment, including specialized radio frequency-energized lighting
- Magnetic separators for capturing metal elements from loose and fragmented materials
- Medical and laboratory devices, such as physiotherapy diathermies, electrical surgery devices, MRI scanners, NMR spectrometers, magnetic therapy devices, and electrical surgery devices
- Power lines and power saws
- Power supply or electric cables of a building
- Power supplying devices, such as high-voltage power lines, transformer stations, and switch yards
- Radio and telecommunication devices, such as radio and television broadcasting antennas and radars
- Resistance welders for connecting metal elements
- Welding equipment
- Wireless or cordless phone systems and base stations

The frequency of EMFs is measured in hertz. Though people are exposed to both electric and magnetic fields, scientists are concerned more about magnetic fields. Employees are exposed to high magnetic fields when they work near electric arrangements that make use of electric power. The strength of a magnetic field is governed by design of equipment and current flow.

Health Implications of EMFs: An EMF may directly or indirectly affect the body of an exposed person because of the absorption of field energy by exposed objects and its effect on the human body. Most indirect effects are caused by contact currents, which flow through the body of a person who comes in contact with a metal object with a different electrical potential. The difference of potential results from exposure to EMF. In case of frequencies below 100 kHz, it can increase electrically sensitive tissues, for instance, muscles or nerves, and cause pain. The intensity and spatial distribution of contact currents depend on the:

- Area of contact between the object and human body
- Dimensions of the exposed object, and
- Frequency of the EMF

An EMF may have lethal effects caused by an impact of technical infrastructure, as currents induced by EMFs in devices may interfere with automatic control devices of electrically controlled equipment. The explosion of combustible materials by spark of an induced current can cause fires and explosions. The human body may experience various effects of EMFs, like:

- Direct exposure stimulates the electrically sensitive tissues owing to the current flow directly induced in the body
- EMFs are not generally perceived by human senses
- EMFs can be recognized directly, for instance, in strong magnetic or electric fields of low frequencies, a person may have visual sensations, called magneto- or electro-phosphenes
- Exposure to pulsed microwave fields can cause hearing sensations, known as Frey effect
- Heating of tissues, including serious burns, caused by energy of field absorbed
- Induced or contact currents flowing through the body may interfere with the functioning of active medical implants (such as pacemakers) and mechanical implants in the body
- Rise of temperature in an exposed body

The health consequences of interaction of EMFs with the human body are not yet established. The mechanisms of human interaction with EMF have been listed.

A. **Conventional mechanisms of human interaction with EMF:**
   - Audio effects by thermo-elastic expansion or Frey effect
   - Electroporation
   - Magneto-hydrodynamic effects
   - Skeletal muscle cell and peripheral nerve excitation by membrane depolarisation
   - Resistive heating
   - Synaptic activity modification by membrane polarisation

B. **Recommended mechanism of human interface with EMF:**

- Alteration by cellular membranes
- Ca^{2+} oscillations
- Ion resonance
- Magnetite interactions
- Nuclear magnetic resonance
- Plasmon resonance
- Radical pair mechanism
- Radon decay product attractors
- Soliton mechanism through cell membrane proteins
- Spatial or temporal cellular integration
- Stochastic resonance
- Temperature-mediated modification of membrane ion transport mechanism

Other detrimental effects also appear and considerably decrease working ability. Such effects, related to movement in the high-level static magnetic field, include dizziness, magneto-phosphenes, nausea, metallic taste in the mouth, and difficulty in coordination of eye and hand. Long-term occupational exposure to EMFs may affect health and capability to work. Until now, no studies have talked about the effect of chronic exposure to EMF at high levels. Probable harmful health effects due to EMF exposure include:

- Development of tumours
- Malfunctions of cardiovascular system
- Malfunctions of immunological system
- Malfunctions of nervous system

Preventive Measures: Different methods can be used to reduce or eliminate EMF. These include filtering, grounding, and shielding. The following measures can help in reducing the effects of EMI:

- Keeping away leads from internal circuits as short as possible to reduce inductance
- Keeping separate grounds for analogue and digital circuits
- Segregating circuits from ground
- Using multiple grounding points

5.6 RADIATION AS WORKPLACE HAZARD

Energy that travels through space is known as radiation. Based on the energy of radiated particles, these are broadly classified into two categories:

Ionizing Radiation: Radiation with slightly large amount of energy that can remove tightly bound electrons from the orbit of an atom, causing that atom to become charged or ionised is referred to as ionizing radiation. These radiations are highly penetrating and can easily damage body tissue. The energy released by atoms travels in the form of electromagnetic waves (gamma or X-rays) or particles (neutrons, beta, or alpha). This spontaneous disintegration of atoms is called radioactivity. The excess energy is emitted in the form of ionizing radiation. The few ionizing radiations that are of concern in most radiological work situations are alpha particles, beta particles, gamma rays, and neutron particles. These may exist in various amounts, depending on the exact location and nature of the work.

Gamma Rays (γ): Gamma rays are the energetic waves of electromagnetic spectrum which are produced by radioactive and nuclear processes like radioactive decay or positron annihilation. Gamma rays have wavelengths of less than ten picometers with highest frequency and shortest wave. Gamma radiation is similar to X-rays in that both pass through living materials easily. These rays are similar to light and have much higher energy and can travel a great distance through air or space. Therefore, they are very penetrating and require shielding of concrete or lead plating to stop them. Gamma radiation is considered an external hazard. Gamma radiations are best shielded by very dense materials, such as lead, concrete, or steel. Shielding is often expressed by thicknesses that provide a certain shielding factor, such as a 'half-value layer' (HVL).

X-Rays: X-ray is an electromagnetic wave or photon having no electrical charge. Gamma rays and X-rays are physically identical, the only difference is in the place of origin. X-rays have no charge and no mass, but have a very high penetrating power. X-rays are characterized by their possibility of interacting in a given material. X-rays are produced when a metallic anode is bombarded by very high energy electrons. They are capable of travelling in a vacuum and are not affected by an electromagnetic field. They can propagate without any medium. They can cause photoelectric emissions.

Alpha Particles (α): Alpha particles are emitted during the decay of certain types of radioactive materials. Compared to other types, the alpha particle has a relatively large mass. It consists of two protons and two neurons. These are highly charged particles that are emitted from the nucleus of an unstable atom. Most alpha particles are stopped by a few centimetres of air, a sheet of paper, or the dead layer (outer layer) of skin on our bodies.

Beta Particles (β): The beta particle is an energetic electron emitted during radioactive decay. Compared to an alpha particle, a beta particle is nearly 8,000 times less massive and has half the electrical charge. Beta radiation causes ionization by electrical interactions with atoms which it encounters as it travels. The beta particle has a limited penetrating ability. Its typical range in air is up to about ten feet. Beta particles are easily shielded by relatively thin layers of plastic, glass, aluminium, or wood.

Neutron Particles (n): Neutron radiation consists of neutrons that are ejected from the nuclei of atoms. A neutron has no electrical charge; hence, it does not interact directly with electrons in matter. A direct interaction occurs as the result of a 'collision' between a neutron and the nucleus of an atom. A charged particle or other radiation which can cause ionization may be emitted during these interactions. This is called indirect ionization. Neutrons have a relatively high penetrating ability and are difficult to stop. Moderate to low energy neutron radiation is best shielded by materials with a high hydrogen content, such as water (H_2O) or polyethylene plastic (CH_2-CH_2-X).

Non-Ionizing Radiation: Non-ionizing radiation is described as a series of energy waves composed of oscillating electric and magnetic fields traveling at the speed of light. Ionization is not caused by these radiations. They usually emit heat, which at times can be so intense and can cause burns. Examples of non-ionizing radiation are ultraviolet rays, microwaves and visible light.

Ultraviolet Rays: Ultraviolet rays have a shorter wavelength when compared with visible light and so we are not able to see in our naked eyes. Ultraviolet rays are present in wavelengths ranging from around 10 nm to around 400 nm. UV radiation is divided into four regions, i.e. near (400–300 nm), middle (300–200 nm), far (200–100 nm), and extreme (below 100 nm). Three types of UV radiations have been classified accordingly in respect to their wavelength. On the interaction of ultraviolet radiation wavelength with biological materials, these are of three types, i.e. UV-A (400 – 315 nm), UV-B (315 – 280 nm), and UV-C (280 – 100 nm). Most solar UV-B is filtered by the atmospheric layer. UV levels are higher when it is closer to the equator.

Visible Light: This part of the electromagnetic spectrum can be seen and distinguished optically by the human eye. Visible light has a wavelength around 400 nm to 700 nm. The white light is a combination of various colours where every colour can be connected with a particular wavelength of light. When white light is passed through a prism, it spreads into the seven colours of the visible light spectrum. These seven colours are Violet, Indigo, Blue, Green, Yellow, Orange, and Red. The visible spectrum in the electromagnetic spectrum ranges from the IR region to the UV region.

Microwaves: Microwaves are high-frequency radio waves and part of the electromagnetic spectrum. Microwaves are reflected, transmitted, or absorbed by materials in their path in a similar manner to visible light. Microwaves are used primarily for TV broadcasting, radar for air and sea navigational aids, and telecommunications including mobile phones. They are also used in industry for processing materials, in medicine for diathermy treatment, and in kitchens for cooking food. Metallic materials completely reflect microwaves while non-metallic materials such as glass and some plastics are generally transparent to microwaves.

Infrared Rays: Infrared rays are electromagnetic radiations with wavelengths longer than those of visible light. Infrared radiation wavelength varies from 700 nanometres to 1 millimetre. Most of the thermal radiation emitted by objects near room temperature is infrared. Depending on the wavelength and frequency, infrared is commonly divided into five categories: near-wavelength, short-wavelength, mid-wavelength, long-wavelength, and far-infrared. Infrared waves are also called heat or thermal waves for they have a particular heat-inducing property. Hot objects and molecules produce infrared waves. Infrared rays are used extensively in remote sensing.

Radio waves: Radio waves are the building block of radio communications with the longest wavelength and lowest frequency in the electromagnetic spectrum. Radio waves are produced naturally by lightning or astronomical objects. Like other electromagnetic radiations, radio waves travel at the speed of light in a vacuum. A radio wave is generated by a transmitter and then detected by a receiver.

Sources of Radiation: The major sources of radiation are:

Cosmic Radiations: Cosmic rays containing highly energetic particles reach the surface of the Earth. Alpha particles, Beta particles, X-rays, and Gamma rays are part of cosmic rays and can damage the human body. The intensity is minimum at the equator and maximum at the poles.

Meteors/Meteorites: Celestial rocks like meteors or meteorites are a source of radioactive metals. When meteors strike the Earth's surface, they release a large amount of radiations to the surrounding environment.

Radioactive Decay: Radioactive decay is the process by which an unstable atomic nucleus loses energy in the form of radiation.

Radioactive Elements: Radioactive elements are made up of atoms having unstable nuclei and during the process of attaining stability release atomic radiation. Minerals containing Uranium-235, Thorium-232, and Plutonium-239 are capable of emitting energetic radiations. The unstable radionuclides in the atmosphere can be split into smaller parts emitting energetic radiation.

Terrestrial Radiation: Natural sources of terrestrial radiation are in the ground, rocks, building materials, and drinking water supplies. Some of the contributors to terrestrial sources are natural radium, uranium, and thorium.

Internal Sources: Our bodies also contain natural radionuclides like Potassium-40.

Anthropogenic Sources: The difference between man-made sources of radiation and naturally occurring sources is the place from which the radiation originates. The following are some examples of human-made radiation sources:

- **Nuclear Weapons and Nuclear Tests:** The nuclear weapon also releases radiation into the environment during testing and the radioactive element contaminates exposed biotic and abiotic components.

- **Consumer Products:** The dose is relatively small as compared to other naturally occurring sources of radiation. TVs, older luminous dial watches, smoke detectors, and lantern mantels are a few examples.
- **Industrial Uses:** Industrial uses of radiation include X-ray machines and radioactive sources (radiography) used to test pipe welds, bore holes, etc.
- **Medical Radiation sources:** X-rays are identical to gamma rays; however, they originate outside the nucleus. X-rays are an ionizing radiation hazard. In addition to X-rays, radioactive isotopes are used in medicine for diagnosis and therapy. Radiation therapy is a cancer treatment that uses high doses of radiation to kill cancer cells and shrink tumours. At low doses, X-rays are used to see broken bones.
- **Nuclear Accidents:** During a nuclear accident, a large number of radionuclides are generated in the atmosphere. These radionuclides settle down with rain contaminating the soil and water bodies. Finally, these enter the food chain, causing serious problem to living organisms.
- **Nuclear Power Plant:** A small amount of radiation is released by nuclear power plants.
- **Nuclear Waste:** Nuclear power plants produce a lot of nuclear radioactive wastes. This waste is source of radioactive elements that release a huge amount of radiation.

Route of Exposure: The route of exposure includes direct or external exposure, inhalation, and ingestion. X-ray is an example of direct exposure. Radon may be inhaled as a gas or ingested if it is in drinking water. Understanding the type of radiation received, the way a person is exposed, and the duration a person is exposed are important in estimating health effects. The risk from exposure to a particular radionuclide depends on the:

- Energy of the radiation it emits
- Type of radiation (alpha, beta, gamma, X-rays)
- Its action, i.e. how often it emits radiation
- Whether the exposure is external or internal:
  - External exposure (when the radioactive source is outside the body. X-rays and gamma rays can pass through the body)
  - Internal exposure (when radioactive material gets inside the body through inhalation, ingestion, or dermal absorption during certain medical procedures). Radionuclides may pose a serious health threat if a substantial amount is inhaled or ingested
- The rate at which the body processes and removes the radionuclide after consumption or breathing
- Site where the radionuclide accumulates in the body and the duration for which it stays inside

Health Implications of Radiation: Based on the dose of radiation received, exposure to radiation may damage living tissues and organs. The extent of probable damage depends on several factors, including the:

- Features of the exposed person (such as age, gender, and well-being)
- Isotopes involved
- Radiation type
- Sensitivity of exposed tissues and organs
- Mode and duration of exposure

Gamma rays have sufficient energy to ionize matter and therefore can damage living cells. The damage produced in the cell or tissue is proportional to the number of ionizing paths produced in the absorbing material. Unshielded gamma rays are harmful inside and outside the body while X-rays have a lower energy than gamma rays but are similar in nature to light. Gamma rays can easily penetrate skin when compared to bone. Due to the high penetrating power, gamma radiation can result in radiation exposure to the whole body rather than a small area of tissue near the source. Likewise, X-rays travel through the air and come in contact with the body tissues, and produce an image on a metal film. Alpha particles are not considered an external radiation hazard for they are easily stopped by the dead layer of skin. If an alpha-emitting radioactive material is inhaled or ingested, it becomes a source of internal exposure. Internally, the source of the alpha radiation is in close contact with body tissue and can deposit large amounts of energy in a small volume of body tissue.

In human tissue, beta particles travel only a few millimetres. Beta particles are potentially hazardous to the skin and eyes. They cannot penetrate to deep tissue such as the bone marrow or other internal organs. When taken into the body, materials that emit beta radiation can be a hazard in a similar way to that described for alpha emitters although comparatively less damage is done in the tissue exposed to the beta emitter. Like gamma radiation, neutrons can cause 'whole body hazard' due to their high penetrating ability.

UV rays differ in their biological activity, and the extent to which they can penetrate the skin. The shorter the wavelength of light, the more harmful the UV radiation will be. However, a shorter wavelength UV radiation is less able to penetrate the skin. Short wavelength UV-C is certainly the most damaging lot of UV radiation. However, it is completely filtered by the atmosphere, and it does not reach the surface of the Earth generally. UV-B is very biologically active but it cannot penetrate beyond the superficial layers of the skin. It is responsible for delayed tanning, and burning of the skin.

The possibility of developing harmful health implications depends on the radiation dose. The higher the dose, the higher will be the risk of damaging effects. If the radiation dose is low or it is delivered for a longer duration, the risk is considerably low for the damage to cells and molecules will be mended by the body.

Acute Health Effects of Radiations: High doses of radiation can impair the functioning of tissues and organs and produce acute effects such as:

- Acute radiation syndrome
- Death
- Hair loss

- Nausea and vomiting
- Radiation burns
- Redness of skin

In a radiological or nuclear disaster, first responders are workers of the nuclear power plant who are at a higher risk for they are exposed to a high dose of radiation which can cause acute effects. A very high dose of radiation exposure delivered over a short period of time can cause acute radiation syndrome, commonly known as '*radiation sickness*'. Acute radiation syndrome is caused when the dose is more than 0.75 gray (75 rad) and duration of exposure is very short, maybe minutes to hours. Acute radiation syndrome is rare, and occurs in extreme events like a nuclear explosion or accidental handling of a highly radioactive source.

Chronic Health Effects of Radiations: Exposure to radiation for a longer duration increases the risk of cancer. Radioactive iodine is released during nuclear emergencies, which if inhaled or absorbed will accumulate in the thyroid gland and increase the risk of thyroid cancer. Moreover, radiation can damage the DNA of cells. High doses of radiation can cause Acute Radiation Syndrome (ARS) or Cutaneous Radiation Injuries (CRI). High doses of radiation can cause cancer. Exposure to low radiation dose does not cause immediate health effects, but increases the risk of cancer.

Like with other pollutants or toxins, the genetic material or DNA, is the primary target. Radiation can directly interact with DNA and damage it by breaking bonds in the DNA. Indirectly it breaks water molecules surrounding the DNA. Once the water molecules break, they produce free radicals – unstable oxygen molecules which can damage cells and organs. Once a cell is impaired, the following can happen:

1. The cell repairs itself and goes back to normal.
2. The cell damage is not repaired or is incorrectly repaired, hence it is changed. This change may ultimately lead to cancer.
3. The cell is damaged to an extent that it dies. If a few radiation-damaged cells die, the body will recover and there will be no risk of those cells possibly turning into cancer. But, extensive cell death, for example caused by high radiation dose, can lead to organ failure and, eventually, death.

Preventive Measures: The aim of radiation protection is to safeguard people and environment against the detrimental effects of ionizing radiation. This is realized through a process called risk assessment which involves:

- Assessing the risk size
- Evaluating its significance in association with other threats
- Identification of potential hazard

The consequences of the risk assessment must be recorded properly and used as the basis for taking decisions in managing the risk. Ultimately, each risk assessment needs to be revised and renewed occasionally and when new apparatus or work practices are introduced.

5.7 HEAT AS WORKPLACE HAZARD

The following four environmental factors affect the stress level a worker has to face in a hot work area:

- Humidity
- Radiant heat (from the sun or a furnace)
- Temperature
- Wind speed

Individuals with high blood pressure (BP) or some heart ailments and people who take diuretics are more sensitive to heat exposure. The body shields itself from heat through three mechanisms, viz.:

- Breathing
- Changing blood flow
- Perspiration

The first response is to disseminate blood to the skin, which increases skin temperature and lets the body emit heat. During heavy work, muscles require more blood flow, which decreases the amount of blood to flow through the skin and discharge heat. Perspiration helps the body to cool off, but only when the humidity level is low enough to allow sweat to vanish and if water and salts lost through perspiration are substituted.

Heat Stress Disorders: When the body overheats, heat stress occurs, which can lead to numerous problems, viz.:

- Fainting
- Heat cramps
- Heat exhaustion
- Heat rash
- Heat stroke

Fainting: It happens when a person is not comfortable working in a hot environment and merely stands. Instead of standing still, moving around generally reduces the chance of fainting.

Symptoms: The symptoms include short-term loss of consciousness, perspiring skin, and normal body temperature, without any signs of heat stroke or heat fatigue. Lying down in a cool place can help in speedy recovery; if not recovered after brief period of lying down medical help can be sought.

Heat Cramps: These are aching, tender muscle spasms, which occur when a worker drinks a lot of water, but does not substitute salts lost from perspiring. Fatigued muscles – those used for executing the work – are generally more likely to have the cramps.

Symptoms: Muscle cramps or spasms may occur during or after the work. Giving electrolyte solution and fluids can relieve the victim.

Heat Exhaustion: It is the most common heat-related ailment that occurs when a worker perspires more and doesn't consume enough fluids or salt or both, which makes the worker wet, white, and weak.

Symptoms: Sweat, feeling weak or tired, perhaps lightheaded, nausea, normal or marginally higher body temperature, pale, sweaty skin.

Heat Rash: It is also known as prickly heat, which occurs in a hot and humid environment and sweat cannot vaporize easily. Later, the rash spreads in a large area or if it gets infected, it may become very painful. Heat rash may be avoided by resting in a cool place and letting the skin dry.

Symptoms: Rash is characterized by small pink or red bumps, with prickly and itching sensation. The condition can be treated by keeping the skin clean and dry to prevent infection, wearing loose cotton clothing, cool baths, and air conditioning, and applying lotions to ease pain and itching.

Heat Stroke: It is the most serious health problem faced by workers working in warm rooms. It is caused when the body fails to control its temperature. During heat stroke sweating stops and the body cannot dispose of excessive heat. Victims may die if not given proper treatment immediately.

Symptoms: Mental confusion, hallucination, collapsing, or seizures, body temperature may reach 106° F or higher. The skin becomes hot, dry, and generally red or bluish colour. This condition calls for medical intervention. Shifting the victim to a cool area and soaking the victim with cool water can help in recovery together with vigorous cooling.

Managing Heat Stress: In most cases, heat stress can be prevented or, at least, the risk of developing heat stress can be reduced.

Engineering Measures: A number of engineering control measures can reduce heat exposure. These are:

- local exhaust ventilation in high heat zones
- removing steam leakages
- safeguarding from radiant heat sources, such as kilns
- using cooling fans or personal cooling gadgets
- using power tools to relieve manual labour

Altering Work Practices

- Consuming plenty of fluids, if the colour of urine is dark yellow, can replace the fluids lost from perspiration. Sports drinks are suggested.
- Employees and labourers returning after an absence of two or more weeks need five days to get acclimatized to heat. Starting with 50 percent of normal workload and less exposure on first day, gradually boost the capacity to 100 percent on the fifth day.
- Heavy work should preferably be planned during the cooler time of the day. When the temperature/humidity index is high, duration of working in hot conditions must be minimized.
- Labour may be at a risk of heat stress if they lose more than 1.5 percent of their body weight in a single day from sweating.
- Wearing loose, light clothing, such as cotton, allows sweat to evaporate. Light colours absorb less heat than dark colours. Wearing a hat keeps the sun off the head and face.

Personal Protective Equipment (PPE): Personal cooling practices, techniques, and devices may reduce the threat of heat stress. Using heat reflective clothing, cooling vest, and liquid cooling systems removes heat from the skin and may lessen the problem of radiant heat sources, such as kilns. Training of workers and administrators can help them in:

- detecting early signs of heat stress
- recognizing the signs of dehydration, fainting, heat cramps, heat exhaustion, and heat stroke
- understanding the need to replace fluids and salt from sweat

Managers must also confirm that the work schedule lets proper rest periods. Labour must use appropriate engineering control measures, PPE, and work practices to reduce the risk of heat stress.

5.8 COLD ENVIRONMENT AS WORKPLACE HAZARD

Anyone working in a cold environment may be at risk of developing health problems. But, older people are at more risk than younger adults, since they are not able to generate heat or regulate body temperature. Some of the health conditions resultant of working in a cold environment are:

Hypothermia or the 'low heat' is a potentially severe health condition which occurs when the body loses heat faster than it can be substituted after being in a cold environment. Symptoms appear with shivering. With falling body temperature, speech becomes inaudible, and the victim lacks coordination and develops memory loss. If the body temperature falls to around 85° F, the person may become unconscious, and at 78° F, the person could die. Some medicines like anti-depressants, sedatives, tranquilizers, and some heart medications may prevent the body from generating heat normally.

Signs and Symptoms

Mild Hypothermia

- inaudible speech
- lack of coordination, stumbling, dropping hands
- pale, cold skin
- quivering

Moderate Hypothermia

- decreased respiration and/or heart rate
- disoriented and illogical
- incapable of standing or walking
- mental confusion or impairment
- shivering ends

Severe Hypothermia

- difficult to find pulse
- drowsy or unconscious
- muscle stiffness
- very cold skin

Mitigation Measures: Proper treatment depends on the severity of hypothermia.

Mild Hypothermia can be handled by avoiding caffeinated beverages and alcohol, consuming warm sugary drinks such as sports drinks, shifting to warm area, removing wet clothes and replacing them with dry clothes or blankets, covering the head, and staying active.

Moderate Hypothermia can be managed by totally **c**overing all the extremities and keeping warm objects, like hot water bottles on victim's head, neck, chest, and groin.

Severe Hypothermia requires careful handling for abrupt movement or rough handling can upset heart rhythms.

Frostbite: Frostbite is another health implication of working in cold climatic condition and occurs when layers of skin tissue freeze. It is caused by exposure to severe cold or by contact with extremely cold objects. In reality, it occurs more speedily from touching cold metal objects because heat is quickly transferred from skin to metal. Frostbite usually affects the extremities, mainly the face, ears, fingers, and toes. Once damaged, tissues become more susceptible to frostbite in the future. In severe cases, amputation of frostbitten area may be required.

Signs and Symptoms include cold, tickling, hurtful or painful feeling in the affected area, followed by numbness, hard or blistered skin which turns red, purple, white, or very pale and is cold to the touch.

Mitigation Measures: By avoiding the rubbing of the affected area, wrapping in a soft cloth can help in overcoming the problem. Dipping in warm water can make the tissue warm.

Cold Stress/Trench Foot or immersion foot: This condition is caused by keeping the feet submerged in cold water for long time. It is alike frostbite, but considered less severe. According to the National Institute for Occupational Safety and Health, cold stress is a condition that appears when the body can no longer maintain its normal temperature. This includes serious injuries resulting in permanent tissue damage or death. Four factors contribute to cold stress: cold temperatures, high or cold wind, dampness, and cold water.

The symptoms include reddening skin, tingling, pain, swelling, leg cramps, numbness, and blisters.

Mitigation Measures: Soaking feet in warm water and wrapping with dry cloth bandages and giving a warm, sugary drink to the victim can accelerate the recovery. Proper planning and wearing appropriate clothing at the workplace in cold weather are the most important defences. Avoiding alcohol and smoking, certain drugs can also help to diminish the risk. Wearing the right clothing is the most important way to avoid cold stress. The type of fabric also makes a difference. Cotton loses its insulation value when it becomes wet. Wool, on the other hand, holds its insulation even when wet. The following work practices can help in reducing the effects of cold-related workplace hazards:

- Drinking plenty of liquids, avoiding caffeine and alcohol
- Scheduling heavy work during the warmer hours of the day
- Working in pairs can help in keeping an eye on each other

Engineering Controls: Following engineering controls can reduce the risk of cold stress:

- Radiant heaters to warm workers and shielding the working areas from winds
- Using insulating material on equipment if the temperature drops below 30° F.

Training: Workers and supervisors must be trained to detect early signs of cold stress. Managers must observe for signs of cold stress. Managers must ensure that work schedules permit suitable rest periods and confirm that plenty of fluids are available. The workplace must adhere to use of suitable engineering controls, PPE, and work practices to moderate the risk of cold stress.

5.9 POOR LIGHTING AS WORKPLACE HAZARD

Appropriate light, without shimmering or darkness, is important for workers who work inside factories, for it reduces eye fatigue and headaches. Working in proper light makes the workers visualize the moving machinery and avert hazards. It decreases the risk of mishaps and injuries from '*temporary impaired vision*' while the eyes acclimatize to brighter or darker environments. The capacity to observe and visualize at the workplace depends not only on proper lighting but on:

Timing: The timing to focus on an object because it is difficult to see fast moving objects

Size: The size of an object for it is difficult to see small objects

Brightness: It is difficult to see in reflected light that is too high or too low

Contrast: It is difficult to distinguish an object from the background and it requires proper contrasting background to notice any object

It is important to take into account and avoid the following at the workplace:

- Blind spot
- Flicker poor lighting
- Glare – too much light
- Improper contrast
- Insufficient light
- Poorly dispersed light
- Thermal heating

Poor lighting can cause several problems such as:

- Affects the quality of work, mainly when accuracy is required
- Health hazard – light that is too high or too low strains the eyes resulting in eye irritation and headaches
- Misjudgement of the position, shape, or speed of an object can cause mishaps and injury

Workers encounter diverse types of light:

Daylight: The amount and direction of sunlight, cloud cover, local terrain, and the season governs the extent of daylight that reaches inside a building. Likewise, the size, alignment, and cleanliness of the windows are also significant. Stained glass, window screens, curtains, and sunshades also control the amount of daylight entering a workplace. Daylight is required in the workplace only if it does not produce glare or make the work area too bright. Not having enough light is also a problem so even in workplaces where daylight is present, it is important to have a suitable and sound electric lighting system.

Electric lighting: The type of electric lighting, amount of light, and colour of light must match the workplace and activities undertaken. There are three basic types of lighting, viz. general, localised-general and local, or task.

Effects of Poor Lighting at Workplace: Proper lighting at the workplace is essential for it can turn out to be a safety or health hazard as well and can cause:

Eye strain: Poor lighting usually leaves the workers with eye strain, which is a very uncomfortable feeling. It can also get linked with other eye-related problems. Spending more time working in poor lighting affects the vision, especially in workplaces that involve working with computers. Setting the contrast and brightness of the computer screen can help in escaping eye strain due to poor lighting. Shifting the table near windows can help in receiving natural light on the work table.

Headache: It is one of the common effects of poor lighting at the workplace which reduces a worker's efficiency. To avoid headaches because of poor lighting, use of desk lamps or computer lamp to brighten up the working area can help in overcoming the problem.

Posture: Poor lighting while working generally makes one sit in an awkward position, resulting in painful back and neck, which can fade away by stretching and yoga.

Low Output: Precision during work depends on light. Poor lighting can result in high chance of human errors. Low precision reduces efficiency which has a direct impact on output.

Accidents: These are hazardous effects of poor lighting at the workplace for it becomes difficult to assess the shape, size, or depth of space or objects. It is often said '*Poor lighting is safety and health hazard*'.

General Well-being: Poor lighting at a workstation makes an employee feel lethargic, dejected, and traumatic. It affects the concentration level and ultimately affects the satisfaction level and has a negative toll on performance. Proper lighting helps improve work efficiency and creates a positive working environment. Consultants or experts can be engaged for light assessment; they can give an idea about the current scenario at your workplace and help in avoiding the effects of poor lighting.

Mitigation Measures: These involve:

- avoiding glare, shadows
- complete use of daylight in the workplace
- ensuring regular cleaning and maintenance of lights and windows
- opting for appropriate visual backgrounds for walls, ceilings, lighting devices and fixtures, etc.

Glare can be reduced from windows by:

- using blinds, curtains, or shades
- replacing clear glass with opaque/translucent materials
- changing the layout of workstations

Glare can be reduced from lamps by:

- ensuring that naked lights are not in direct view of workers
- ensuring that the working area is well lit
- using shades or shields

Glare can be reduced from reflected glare by:

- changing the position of light source and reducing its brightness
- changing the layout of the workstations
- covering reflecting surface with opaque, non-glossy material

5.10 ERGONOMIC HAZARDS

Ergonomic hazards are physical situations that may pose a hazard of injury to the musculoskeletal system because of poor ergonomics. These hazards include:

- Awkward or prolonged/static postures
- Carrying
- Contact stress
- Force
- Gripping
- Heavy lifting
- High forces
- Overhead work
- Push or pull
- Repetitive motion or short intervals between activities
- Vibration

The risk of injury is often enlarged when multiple factors exist. Environmental, operational, or design factors can have a negative impact on workers or users; examples include:

- Badly designed tools, equipment, or workstations
- Inadequate lighting
- Whole-body or hand/arm vibration

Some common body areas likely to get injured may include:

- Bones and muscles surrounding the knees and legs
- Muscles or ligaments of neck
- Muscles or ligaments of lower back
- Muscles, tendons, or nerves of hands/wrists

Injuries in other body parts could result in musculoskeletal disorders (MSDs), which may be called cumulative trauma disorders (CTDs) or repetitive strain injuries (RSIs), and are estimated to account for about one-third of all non-fatal injuries and illnesses and their associated costs. Ergonomic hazards occur in both occupational and non-occupational settings such as:

- Building sites
- Homes
- Offices
- Public spaces and facilities
- Schools
- Workshops

Finding methods to reduce or reduce ergonomic hazards in any situation will eventually decrease the risk of injury.

Musculoskeletal Disorders or MSDs: These are cumulative and chronic injuries of:

- Blood vessels
- Discs
- Joints
- Ligaments
- Nerves
- Soft tissue-muscles
- Tendons

MSDs are caused or intensified by body actions and/or environment or not following safe and healthy work practices. A well-known MSD is carpal tunnel syndrome which occurs when the nerve, which runs from the forearm into the palm of the hand, becomes pressed or squeezed at the wrist.

Symptoms of MSDs: The main symptoms include:

- Burning sensation
- Clumsiness
- Debility
- Discomfort
- Rigidity
- Sensitivity
- Sleepiness
- Swelling
- Tickling
- Trouble in moving

Ergonomic Risk Factors: Ergonomic risk factors are workplace situations that cause wear and tear on the body and can cause injury. Multiple factors that increase the risks of developing MSD are:

1. **Direct Pressure:** Direct pressure is the resultant of prolonged contact of body with a hard or sharp surface or edge that prevents nerve function and limits the blood flow. This may include contact with desk edges or unpadded, narrow tool handles.
2. **Excessive Noise:** Exposure to excessive noise occurs in the following workplaces:
   - Bars and clubs
   - Construction
   - Manufacturing
   - Mining
   - Processing

   Excessive noises such as those caused by explosions can cause permanent hearing loss.

3. **Excessive Vibration:** The use of vibrating tools in manufacturing and construction, and other industries, is the most common cause of vibration-related hazards. This damage can lead to reduced blood flow, smashed nerves, and muscle weariness.
4. **Extreme Temperatures:** Extreme temperatures (hot or cold) are severe ergonomic hazards. Intense cold leads to hypothermia and frostbite, affects motor coordination and dexterity, affecting workers to use great force to execute tasks. Extreme heat can cause heat stroke. Outdoor workers are more at risk of temperature-related ergonomic hazards.
5. **Forceful Motions:** This ergonomic hazard occurs when unnecessary effort is required to complete tasks. It can include pulling, pounding, pushing, and lifting which can affect the tendons, joints, and discs and can cause irritation, inflammation and constriction of blood vessels or nerves. Forceful motion hazards are more common in manufacturing and construction.
6. **Recurrent Lifting:** Heavy lifting can cause muscle strain and is a recurrent source of injuries to workers. An object's weight, distribution, shape, and location relative to the body, play a role in the gravity of this hazard. Back problems are the most common result of both heavy and frequent lifting, mainly if it is done inaccurately.
7. **Improper Lighting:** Insufficient lighting in a store, industrial unit, or office can result in accidents and injuries. It can also strain eyes, triggering discomfort and headaches. Glare affects a worker's ability to clearly see objects and lead to pain and impaired vision. Inappropriately dispersed light is also a glitch at workplaces, where the amount of light varies considerably from space to space, compelling workers to adjust their vision constantly.
8. **Poor Posture:** Poor posture is another common ergonomic hazard. It also upsets workers in manufacturing units involving standing or sitting for long periods. It is generally the result of badly placed

devices that may require a worker to lean forward or reach uncomfortably to get them. A poorly designed chair or stool also results in problematic posture.

9. **Repetitive Motions:** Repetitive motion injuries are the most common type of injury in the workplace. This hazard is the result of a worker making the same motion, over and over again, for extended periods of time. It can occur in industries involved in packing, assembling, typing, welding or even sweeping.
10. **Stationary Positions:** Continuing in one position for a long duration can restrict blood flow and cause fatigue and damage the muscles and joints. It is a common cause of leg, neck, and back pain. Awkward position stresses the spine. Workers having sedentary jobs must be aware of the hazards that are common in sedentary jobs for long duration.

Mitigating Ergonomic Risks: It involves:

- Identification is the first step in addressing ergonomic hazards.
- Once the risks are identified, these can be addressed. Many injuries caused by ergonomic hazards are cumulative in nature; hence, their early detection is vital.
- The mitigating measures for ergonomic hazards include:
  - designing workstations for reducing awkward positions
  - following strict protocols for performing tasks
  - frequent rest breaks, changes in position or duties
  - providing appropriate personal protective equipment (PPE) and work attire
  - replacing the more repetitive and difficult actions performed by workers by using robotic equipment
  - using modern tools for mitigating or reducing excessive vibrations, noise, pressure, or force

Engineering Improvements: These include reorganizing, amending, reshaping, or substituting tools, equipment, workplaces, packaging, parts, or products.

Administrative Improvements: These include changing work practices or the way work is planned, viz.:

- Regulating work schedules and work pace
- Encouraging exercise, personal protective equipment, use of safety gears
- Confirming regular housekeeping and maintenance of work spaces, tools, and equipment
- Amending work practices
- Offering diversity in jobs
- Providing recovery time (i.e. muscle relaxation time)

BIBLIOGRAPHY

(1985) Identification and Control of Work-Related Diseases. Report Series 714. Geneva, Switzerland: World Health Organization.

Anderson, J. A. D. (1984) Shoulder pain and tension neck and their relation to work. Scandinavian Journal of Work, Environment, and Health 19(6):435–442.

Arad, D. and Ryan, M. D. (1986) The incidence and prevalence in nurses of low back pain. Australian Nurses Journal 16:44–48.

Ariens, G. A. M., Mechelen, W., van, Bongers, P. M., Bouter, L. M. and Wal, G. van der (2000) Physical risk factors for neck pain. Scandinavian Journal of Work, Environment, and Health 26:7–19.

Armstrong, T. J., Fine, L. J., Radwin, R. G. and Silverstein, B. S. (1987) Ergonomics and the effects of vibration in hand-intensive work. Scandinavian Journal of Work, Environment, and Health 13:286–289.

Baidya, K. N. and Stevenson, M. G. (1988) Local muscle fatigue in repetitive work. Ergonomics 31:227–239.

Baum, A. and Posluszny, D. M. (1999) Health psychology: Mapping behavioural contributions to health and illness. Annual Review of Psychology 50:137–163.

Bayley, J. (1991) Health and safety at work. British Dental Journal 170(10):364–365.

Bergenuud, H. and Nilsson, B. (1988) Occupational workload and psychologic factors: An epidemiologic survey. Spine 13:58–60.

Biem, J., Koehncke, N., Classen, D. and Dosman, J. (2003) Out of the cold: Management of hypothermia and frostbite. CMAJ 168:305–311.

Brake, D. J. and Bates, G. P. (2002) Deep body core temperatures in industrial workers under thermal stress. Journal of Occupational and Environmental Medicine 44:125–135.

Brake, D. J. and Bates, G. P. (2002) Deep body core temperatures in industrial workers under thermal stress. Journal of Occupational and Environmental Medicine 44:125–135.

Bru, E. and Mykletun, R. J. (1996) Work related stress and musculoskeletal pain among female hospital staff. Work and Stress 10(4):309–321.

Cohen, R. (1990) Injuries due to physical hazards. In Occupational Medicine (Ladou, J. ed.). USA: Prentice-Hall International, Inc.

Conway, H. and Svenson, J. (1998) Occupational injury and illness rates, 1992-96: Why they fell. Monthly Labor Review 121(11):36–58.

Cutler, R. (1991) Health and safety at work. British Dental Journal 170(7):251.

Dash, S. K. and Kjellstrom, T. (2011) Workplace heat stress in the context of rising temperature in India. Current Science 101:496–503.

David, G. (2005) Ergonomic methods for assessing exposure to risk factors for work-related musculoskeletal disorders. Occupational Medicine 55(3):190–199.

Enander, A. (1984) Performance and sensory aspects of work in cold environments: A review. Ergonomics 27:365–378.

Hernberg, S. (1992) Introduction to Occupational Epidemiology. Philadelphia: Lewis Publishers.

Kim, J. Y., Jung, K. Y., Hong, Y. S., Kim, J. I., Jang, T. W. and Kim, J. M. (2003) The relationship between cold exposure and hypertension. Industrial Health 45:300–306.

Levy, B. S. and Wegman, D. H. (1994) Occupational Health: Recognizing and Preventing Work-Related Disease. Boston: Little Brown.

NIOSH. (1996) National Occupational Research Agenda. Publication No. 96-115. U.S. Department of Health and Human Services, Public Health Service, Centers for Disease Control and Prevention, National Institute for Occupational Safety and Health. Washington, DC: U.S. Department of Health and Human Services.

Nichols, T. (1998) Health and safety at work. Work, Employment & Society 12(2):367–374.

(2000) OSHA3125, Ergonomics: The Study of Work. U.S. Department of Labor Occupational Safety and Health Administration.

Parsons K. (2002) Human Thermal Environments: The Effects of Hot, Moderate and Cold Environments on Human Health, Comfort and Performance. New York: CRC Press.

Pilcher, J. J., Nadler, E. and Busch. C. (2002) Effects of hot and cold temperature exposure on performance: A meta-analytic review. Ergonomics 45:682–698.

Rosenstock, L. and Cullen, M. R. (1994) Textbook of Clinical Occupational and Environmental Medicine. Philadelphia: Saunders.

Scott, R. M. (2020) Chemical Hazards in the Workplace (e-book). Boca Raton: CRC Press.

Spurlock, B. (2017) Physical Hazards of the Workplace. Boca Raton: CRC Press.

Wilson, H. G. E. and Agius, R. M. (1994) Health and safety at work. BMJ 309(6948):198–199.

World Health Organization. (1977) World Health Classification: Manual of the International Statistical Classification of Diseases, Injuries, and Causes of Death. 9th Revision. Geneva, Switzerland: World Health Organization.

Wyon, D. P., Kok, R., Lewis, M. I. and Meese, G. B. (1982) The effects of moderate cold and heat stress on factory workers in Southern Africa: Introduction to a series of full-scale simulation studies. South African Journal of Science 78:184–189.

6 Occupational Diseases

"An incident is just the tip of the iceberg, a sign of a much larger problem below the surface"

—Anonymous

FACT FILE

- The International Labour Organization estimates that some 2.3 million people across the globe die due to occupation-related accidents or diseases every year
- Globally, there are around 340 million occupational accidents and 160 million fatalities from work-related illnesses each year
- Work-related diseases cause most deaths among workers and hazardous substances alone cause more than 650,000 deaths per year
- The construction industry has an excessively high rate of recorded accidents
- Younger and older workers are mainly susceptible
- Poor working environs – including prejudice and disparity, unnecessary workloads, low job control, and job uncertainty – pose a threat to mental health
- Worldwide, an approximated 12 billion working days are lost annually to depression and anxiety
- According to the WHO, the majority of work-related deaths are due to respiratory and cardiovascular diseases
- According to the WHO, non-communicable diseases accounted for 81 percent of the deaths
- According to the WHO, the greatest causes of deaths are chronic obstructive pulmonary disease followed by stroke and ischaemic heart disease
- Occupational injuries caused 19 percent of deaths
- Effective actions, viz., promotion of mental health at work, and supporting workers with mental health conditions can help in prevention of mental health risks

6.1 INTRODUCTION

The term *occupational disease* covers any disease developed because of an exposure to risk factors arising from work activity. Occupational illness is any

DOI: 10.1201/9781003464785-6

abnormal condition or disorder, other than one resulting from an occupational injury triggered by exposure to environmental factors linked with occupation or workplace. It can be acute or chronic illnesses, after an exposure to hazards through inhalation, absorption, ingestion, or direct contact. The ILO defines occupational diseases as:

> "… diseases known to arise after exposure to substances and unsafe conditions in procedures, trades or occupations …"

The two main elements in the definition of an occupational disease focus on:

- the causal relationship between exposure in a working environment or work activity and a specific disease; and
- the fact that the disease occurs among a group of exposed persons with a frequency above the average morbidity of the rest of the population.

6.2 STANDARDS FOR CATEGORIZATION AND RECOGNITION OF OCCUPATIONAL DISEASES

The causal relationship between a specific occupational disease and contributing exposure is established on the basis of:

- clinical and pathological data
- occupational background and job analysis
- identification and evaluation of occupational risk factors
- role of other risk factors

Epidemiological and toxicological data is useful for establishing the causal relationship between a specific occupational disease and its causal exposure in a specific working environment. The symptoms are not adequately representative to identify an occupational disease without understanding the pathological changes induced by the physical, chemical, biological, or other factors faced at the workplace. It is therefore normal that, as a result of improvements in knowledge about the mechanisms of action, it becomes more and more realistic to make a precise diagnosis, while the range of diseases spotted as occupational in origin is widening. It depends on:

- **Intensity of association:** The greater the impact of an exposure on the occurrence or development of a disease, the greater is the possibility of an underlying association.
- **Specificity:** Exposure to a specific risk factor results in a clearly defined pattern of diseases.
- **Temporality or time sequence:** The exposure of interest led the disease by a period of time steady with a projected biological mechanism.
- **Biological gradient:** The greater the level and duration of exposure, the greater will be the severity of diseases or its prevalence.

- **Biological credibility:** From what is known of toxicology, chemistry, physical properties, or other features of the investigated risk or hazard, it makes biological sense to recommend that exposure accounts for a disease.
- **Consistency:** A general synthesis of all evidence concludes that there is a cause-effect relationship both in terms of a wider and general practicality.
- **Interventional analyses:** At times, a principal preventative trial may confirm whether eliminating a particular hazard or decreasing a specific risk from the working environment or work activity removes the development of a specific disease or lessens its incidence.

Key fundamentals for determining causal relationships are:

- the exposure-effect relationship (relation between exposure and the severity of the damage in the subject)
- the exposure-response relationship (association between exposure and relative number of subjects affected)

Research and epidemiological studies have significantly added to this field. Better knowledge of the causative association has permitted to achieve a better medical definition of occupational diseases. Consequently, the legal explanation of occupational diseases, which was somewhat problematic, is becoming more and more associated to the medical definition and criteria. However, legal provisions on compensation for victims vary across different nations. The Employment Injury Benefits Convention points out several prospects about the form of identification of Occupational Diseases enabling workers to claim reimbursement benefits. It states that each member shall:

a. suggest a list of diseases, comprising at least the diseases listed in the Convention, which shall be considered as *Occupational Disease* under suggested environments; or
b. include in its regulation a general definition of *Occupational Disease* comprehensive enough to cover at least the diseases detailed in the convention; or
c. recommend a list of diseases in accordance to the clause (a), supplemented by a general definition of *Occupational Disease* or by other provisions for establishing the occupational origin of diseases not so enumerated or demonstrating themselves under conditions different from those prescribed

The List of Occupational Diseases Recommendation, 2002 (No. 194) was accepted at the 90th Session of the International Labour Conference, 2002. The Committee on Occupational Accidents and Diseases established in 2002 to work on the List of Occupational Diseases Recommendation demanded the Governing Body of the International Labour Office to organize the first of the tripartite meetings of experts referred to in the recommendation as a matter of urgency. The Committee expected that, besides scrutinizing the Annex to the Recommendation, the existing national and other lists of occupational diseases, and the observations received from member states, the meeting must ponder on all the modifications submitted on the Annex to the Conference Committee. The occupational diseases can be classified on the following basis:

A. **Occupational Diseases by Target Organ Systems**
   - Occupational Musculo-skeletal disorders
   - Occupational Respiratory diseases
   - Occupational Skin diseases

B. **Occupational Cancer**
   - Cancer caused by various agents

C. **Occupational Diseases Caused by Exposure to Workplace Agents**
   - Diseases caused by Biological agents
   - Diseases caused by Chemical agents
   - Diseases caused by Physical agents

D. **Other Diseases**
   - Miners' nystagmus

6.3 OCCUPATIONAL DISEASES BY TARGET ORGAN SYSTEMS

6.3.1 Respiratory Diseases

Recurrent and long-term exposure to certain irritants at the workplace can cause an array of lung diseases that may have long-lasting effects, even after exposure ceases. Certain professions, owing to the nature of their location, work, and environment, are more at risk for causing occupational lung diseases than others. In contrast to a common fallacy, coal miners are not the only ones at risk for occupational lung diseases; for instance, working in a garage or textile factory can expose a person to harmful substances, dusts, and fibres that may cause a lifetime of lung problems if not identified and cured suitably. Irrespective of the cause, the following are the most common symptoms of lung diseases; but, each individual may experience symptoms in a different way. Signs may include:

- Abnormal breathing pattern
- Chest pain
- Chest tightness
- Coughing
- Shortness of breath

The symptoms of occupational lung diseases may be similar to other medical conditions or problems. A few lung diseases linked with occupation are:

- Aluminosis (also known as aluminium lung) is a restrictive lung disease caused by exposure to aluminium-bearing dust. Aluminosis is a form of pneumoconiosis that can lead to pulmonary fibrosis

- Asthma caused by recognized sensitizing agents or irritants inherent to the work process
- Broncho-pulmonary diseases caused by dust of cotton (byssinosis), flax, hemp, sisal, or sugarcane (bagassosis)
- Broncho-pulmonary diseases caused by hard metal dust
- Chronic obstructive pulmonary diseases caused by inhalation of coal dust, dust from stone quarries, wood dust, dust from cereals and agricultural work, dust in animal stables, dust from textiles, and paper dust, arising from work activities
- Extrinsic allergic alveolitis caused by the inhalation of organic dusts or microbially-contaminated aerosols, released from work activities
- Pneumoconiosis caused by fibrogenic mineral dust (silicosis, anthraco-silicosis, asbestosis)
- Pneumoconiosis caused by non-fibrogenic mineral dust
- Siderosis, a pathological condition of lung caused by long continued inhalation of the dust of iron or iron oxide
- Silico-tuberculosis disease is caused by silica exposure, and is often found in TB endemic countries
- Upper airway disorders due to recognized sensitizing agents or irritants inherent to the work process

6.3.2 Skin Diseases

Exposure to chemical, physical, and biological risk factors can cause different skin diseases, though several individual (genetic) factors also affect the outcome. Occupational skin diseases account for about 50 percent of occupational illnesses. Skin diseases affect workers of all ages in all types of work environments but a majority of diseases are caused by wet work, workplace exposure to chemicals, and high ultraviolet radiation from the sun. In context of skin the most relevant chemical hazards are:

- Acnegenic agents
- Irritant agents
- Photosensitizing agents
- Sensitizing agents

Biological hazards range from bacteria, fungi, and viruses, to skin parasites, while physical hazards include rubbing, mechanical pressure, radiations, and temperature.

- Allergic contact dermatoses and contact urticaria caused by other recognized allergy- provoking agents arising from work activities not included in other items
- Irritant contact dermatoses caused by other recognized irritant agents arising from work activities not included in other items
- Vitiligo caused by other recognized agents arising from work activities not included in other items

6.3.3 Musculoskeletal Disorders

- Radial styloid tenosynovitis attributable to:
  - Extreme postures of the wrist
  - Forceful exertions
  - Repetitive movements
- Chronic tenosynovitis of hand and wrist because of:
  - Extreme postures of the wrist
  - Forceful exertions
  - Repetitive movements
- Olecranon bursitis due to prolonged pressure of the elbow region
- Prepatellar bursitis attributable to prolonged stay in a kneeling position
- Epicondylitis caused by repetitive forceful work
- Meniscus lesions following extended periods of work in a kneeling or squatting position
- Carpal tunnel syndrome as a result of:
  - Extended periods of repetitive forceful work
  - Extreme postures of the wrist,
  - Work involving vibration, or a combination of the three

6.4 MENTAL AND BEHAVIOURAL DISORDERS

Mental disorders in the workplace are a major public health problem. Knowledge of the impact of the psychosocial work environment on mental and behavioural disorders can assist occupational physicians in the identification and description of occupational risk situations, and help to define priority actions.

Post-traumatic stress disorder (PTSD) occurs as a prolonged response to a traumatic incident or condition, either short-term or long-term, of an exceptionally intimidating or terrible nature involving threat to life and safety, such as:

- Civil riots
- Criminal offences
- Environmental disasters
- War events

Thus, the cause of PTSD is any direct or indirect exposure to an enormously threatening or terrible event or series of events. A devastating event is defined as one that is outside the normal range of everyday life events experienced by an individual. It usually involves a threat to one's life. Events and situations causing occupational PTSD include:

- Workplace violence (incidents where staff members are mistreated or assaulted at workplace circumstances that challenge their safety, well-being, or health)
- Physical violence (use of physical force that causes physical, sexual, or psychological harm)

- Psychological violence (emotional abuse harming the physical, mental, spiritual, moral, or social well-being). Such violence includes:
  - Harassment or mobbing
  - Annoyance
  - Terrorizations
  - Public humiliation

The onset of PTSD symptoms has often been noticed in victims of these situations as well.

- **Occupational exposure:** Workplace violence affects many occupations but is more common in an industrial setup. The following are exposed to PTSD symptoms:
  - Ambulance staff, viz. nurses and physicians
  - Clerks in retail establishments
  - Military personnel, and other emergency responders
  - Police officers
  - Security guards
  - Staff at airport ticket counters
  - Ticket takers
  - Urban bus or trolley drivers and conductors
  - Workers engaged in emergency
  - Workers engaged in fire-fighting
  - Workers engaged in rescue
  - Workers in banks and other public institutions
  - Workers in government and private sector

Primary Preventive Measures: These include:

- Collective preparedness and safety measures by taking care of appropriate workplace design, safety precautions, and protective measures
- Description of potential risks
- Effective training on safety precautions for possible traumatic events
- Involvement of workplace occupational health services
- Safety exercises for the events likely to occur
- Training on prevention, avoidance, control, and preparedness
- Training on self-defence and self-protection where appropriate

The secondary prevention measures required depend on the type and context of trauma or event. Acute stress reactions can be handled with the involvement of occupational health personals.

Tertiary Preventive Measures: These involve:

- Early identification of symptoms using clinical criteria
- For acute and short-term reactions (below three months):

- deliver good and reliable relaxing contact and follow-up
- ensure the company of a social network, family, friends, and other social cohorts
- offer an individual trauma-focused cognitive behavioural therapy (CBT)
- offer help and support in routine activities

Tertiary prevention requires access to mental health services. The specific interventions may include:

- engaging with trauma-focused therapies
- follow-up of individuals after traumatic event
- pharmacotherapy for established symptoms taking into account the best practices
- specialized clinical care with cognitive behavioural therapy (CBT)

6.5 OCCUPATIONAL CANCERS

Work-related exposure to chemicals, dusts, radiation, and industrial processes is linked with occupational cancer. Exposure to carcinogens, the cancer-causing chemicals, results in mutations as a result of which the cells grow out of control, causing cancer. The risk factors for cancer include:

- Personal characteristics such as age, gender, and race
- Family background of cancer
- Overweight or obesity
- Diet and personal habits like consumption of tobacco and alcohol
- Certain medical conditions or past medical treatments, including chemotherapy and radiation treatment
- Use of immune-suppressing drugs
- Certain infectious agents, viz. viruses, bacteria, parasites
- Exposure to cancer-causing agents present in the environment, for instance, sunlight, radon gas, air pollution

Asbestos, second hand smoke, and benzene are the main carcinogens that people are commonly exposed to at work. Lung cancer, mesothelioma, bladder cancer, and leukaemia are commonly occurring cancers resultant of occupational exposure to carcinogens. More than 125 million people around the world are exposed to asbestos at work, and at least 90000 die each year from asbestos-related diseases. Besides this, deaths due to lung cancer are closely linked with workplace risks. Thousands of people working in the chemical and diamond industries die from leukaemia after exposure to benzene, which is one of the widely used organic solvents. According to the WHO, prevention of exposure to carcinogens at the workplace may be the most effective way of preventing cancer.

Cancer-causing Agents at workplace include:

1. **Arsenic and its compounds**

Occupational Exposure: Workers involved in the following are exposed to arsenic and its compounds:

- Arsenic containing compounds used in industrial processes meant for production of:
  - fungicides
  - herbicides
  - insecticides
  - wood preservatives
- Manufacturing arsenic containing pigments, bronze articles
- Preparation and manufacturing of alloys
- Production of microelectronics, glassmaking, and optical industry
- Smelting of sulphide-arsenide ores in primary metallurgy

Type of Cancer: Bladder cancer, lung cancer, skin cancer

2. **Asbestos**

Occupational Exposure: Workers involved in the following are exposed to asbestos:

- Fireproofing and thermal insulation of boilers, pipes, industrial reactors, buildings
- Manufacturing lightweight and resistant items for building, especially water pipes and roofing tiles
- Extraction and production of various asbestos products
- Manufacturing products containing asbestos cement like:
  - Acoustic purposes
  - Asbestos paper
  - Clapboards
  - Pipes
  - Shingles
  - Spray products used for thermal, fireproofing
  - Vinyl-asbestos floor tiles
- Textile products such as yarns, tape, cord, rope, and felt
- Occupations potentially linked with asbestos exposure are:
  - Boiler makers
  - Insulation workers
  - Janitors
  - Pipe fitters
  - Plumbers
  - Steamfitters
  - Welders

Type of Cancer: Malignant mesothelioma, lung cancer, laryngeal cancer, ovarian cancer

3. **Benzene**

Occupational Exposure: Workers involved in the following are exposed to benzene:

- benzene production (petrochemicals, petroleum refining, and coke and coal chemical manufacturing)
- chemical industry for synthesis of a great variety of chemical products
- dealing with car fuel
- extraction of natural crude petroleum, coal derivatives and petroleum fractions, and distillates
- extraction of oils from seeds and nuts
- manufacturing detergents, explosives, intermediates for dyes and pharmaceuticals
- production and handling of gasoline fuels
- rubber manufacturing
- storage or transport of benzene

Production and use of solvents and thinners for:

- Adhesives
- Dry cleaning
- Fats
- Glues
- Inks
- Lacquers
- Oils
- Paints
- Plastics
- Resins
- Rubber
- Scouring of metal parts
- Waxes

Occupational exposure is higher among the following:

- Fire-fighters
- Gas station employees
- Laboratory technicians
- Printers
- Shoemakers
- Steelworkers

Type of Cancer: Acute myeloid leukaemia (AML)

4. **Beryllium and its compounds**

Occupational Exposure: Workers involved in the following are exposed to beryllium and its compounds:

- Decommissioning and recycling of items and waste materials
- Metal extraction and refining
- Preparation and machining of its alloys into usable goods by melting, grinding, welding, and drilling
- Recycling of end life manufactured goods for valuable constituents

Type of Cancer: Lung cancer

5. **Cadmium and its compounds**

Occupational Exposure: Workers involved in the following are exposed to cadmium and its compounds:

- Battery manufacturing, electroplating, plastics, ceramics, paint, and welding
- Cadmium fumes are generated in production of cadmium alloys, in welding, and oxyacetylene cutting of cadmium-coated steel
- Manufacturing of colourant for pyrotechnics
- Electroplating of iron and steel, paint pigmentation
- Manufacturing of nickel-cadmium batteries
- Metal machining
- Dyeing
- Printing textiles
- Production of fertilizers
- Smelting and refining of metals
- Stearate heat stabilization in polyvinyl chloride (PVC) plastics

Type of Cancer: Lung cancer

6. **Chromium VI compounds**

Occupational Exposure: Workers involved in several industrial operations linked with manufacturing of:

- Inorganic pigments such as:
    - Lead chromates (to prepare chrome greens)
    - Zinc chromate
    - Molybdate oranges
    - Chromium oxide green

- Corrosion inhibition
- Wood preservation
- Coloured glasses and glazes
- Tanning

Occupational exposure to hexavalent chromium can thus be related to activities such as:

- Chromium coating
- Engraving and lithography
- Fabric dyeing
- Leather tanning
- Manufacturing of batteries
- Painting as anticorrosive pigments in paints
- Stainless steel welding

Type of Cancer: Lung cancer

7. **Coal tars/coal tar pitches/soot**

Occupational Exposure: Workers involved in the following are exposed to coal tar:

- Brick making for household heating
- Coal distillation
- Coke manufacturing
- Coke or coal gas plants
- Operating cheap-fuel in burners
- Roofing activities, viz. removal of an old roof by cutting, prying, and scraping
- Timber proofing
- Wooden railway sleepers and electric wire poles where timber contains preservatives

Workers involved in the following are exposed to soot:

- Blast furnaces
- Chimney sweeping
- Coal or liquid fuel fired power plants
- Coke ovens
- Combustion plants
- Ship engine rooms

Type of Cancer: Skin cancer, lung cancer

8. **Coke oven emissions**

Occupational Exposure: Workers involved in the following are exposed to coke oven emissions:

- Blast furnace plants, during the production of coke from coal
- Carbonization process
- Coal gas plants upstream to production of bulk chemicals
- Inhalation of dusts and vapours
- Reducing agent to make iron and steel in blast furnaces

Type of Cancer: Lung Cancer

9. **Ethylene oxide**

Occupational Exposure: Workers involved in the following are exposed to ethylene oxide:

- agrochemicals manufacturing
- detergents manufacturing
- fumigation of food products, such as packaged cereals, bagged rice, and spices
- maintenance or repair work or are dedicated to cleaning reactors
- manufacturing of pharmaceuticals
- oilfield chemicals and personal care products
- sterilization of surgical equipment
- textile sector

Type of Cancer: Breast cancer, chronic lymphocytic leukaemia (CLL), multiple myeloma (MM), and non-Hodgkin lymphoma (NHL)

10. **Hepatitis B virus (HBV) and Hepatitis C virus (HCV)**

Occupational Exposure: Workers involved in the following are exposed to Hepatitis B virus (HBV):

- Clinical laboratories handling biological specimens
- Contact with infected human blood and body fluids
- Handling sharp injuries, such as needle stick accidents, are the most frequent exposure event
- Health workers
- Police and ambulance crews
- Workers employed in rescue services
- Personal relationships (sexual intercourse, mother-to-child transmission, sharing of personal items, such as shaving razors, scissors, toothbrushes, and needles)

Type of Cancer: Liver cancer (hepatocellular carcinoma), non-Hodgkin lymphoma

11. **Ionizing radiations**

Occupational Exposure: Workers involved in the following are exposed to ionizing radiations:

- Aircrew members: Exposed to cosmic radiation, a form of ionizing radiation coming from outer space
- Activity involving the use of isotopes, uranium, and other mines, any other activity conducted underground and ordinary workplaces in areas that are rich in radon emission.
- Artificial sources of radiation used in the manufacturing, service, and defence industries
- Healthcare activities
- In industry, dealing with particle accelerators, gamma radiography sources, nuclear reactors
- Physicians and health professionals, in the diagnosis and in treatment of diseases
- Research institutions and universities, and in the nuclear power industry

Type of Cancer: Malignant neoplasms, skin cancer, leukaemia, lung cancer, osteosarcoma

12. **Nickel compounds**

Occupational Exposure: Workers involved in the following are exposed to nickel compounds:

- Alloy and stainless steel manufacture
- Electroplating and electroextraction
- Manufacturing of nickel cadmium batteries, coins, and kitchen utensils
- Nickel refinery and nickel smelter workers
- Nickel-producing industries, viz. mining, milling, smelting, and refining, and in nickel-using industries and operations
- Recycling operations especially in the steel industry
- Welding, grinding, and cutting

Type of Cancer: Cancer of the nasal cavity and para-nasal sinuses, lung cancer

13. **Tar, pitch, bitumen, mineral oil, anthracene, or the compounds, products or residues of these substances**

Occupational Exposure: Workers involved in the following are exposed to tar, pitch, bitumen, mineral oil, anthracene, or the compounds, products, or residues of these substances:

- Building roofing
- Industrial chemical plants for tar distillation, coal gas, and asphalt production, cleaning of tankers and raw and refined petroleum spillage, and burning of petroleum
- Insulation
- Newspaper printing

- Protecting metals from air oxidation in processing and manufacturing
- Road paving
- Waterproofing

Type of Cancer: Skin cancer

14. **Toxic nitro- and amino-derivatives of benzene or its homologues**

Occupational Exposure: Workers involved in the following are exposed to toxic nitro- and amino-derivatives of benzene or its homologues:

- Health workers, in particular laboratory and medical personnel
- Polyurethane industry
- Production and use as a dye intermediate or as a rubber antioxidant
- Production of o-toluidine and of dyes, pigments, and rubber chemicals
- Tobacco smoke and the use of some hair dyes

Type of Cancer: Bladder cancer

15. **Vinyl chloride**

Occupational Exposure: Workers involved in the following are exposed to vinyl chloride:

- Manufacturing of industrial chemicals, plastic products, fabricated metal products, and non-electrical machinery
- Manufacturing of polyvinyl chloride (PVC)
- Production and polymerization plants

Type of Cancer: Liver angiosarcoma, hepatocellular carcinoma

16. **Wood dust**

Occupational Exposure: Workers involved in the following activities are exposed to wood dust:

- Cabinet making
- Construction carpentry
- Construction of building fittings
- Inhaled by timber workers, carpenters, and cabinet-makers
- Making of industrial furniture
- Model making
- Sawing, milling, sanding of wood
- Wooden boat manufacture
- Woodwork

Type of Cancer: Cancer of nasal cavity, paranasal sinuses, nasopharynx

6.6 OCCUPATIONAL DISEASES CAUSED BY EXPOSURE TO WORKPLACE AGENTS

6.6.1 Diseases Caused by Biological Agents

Anthrax: It is an infection caused by the bacterium *Bacillus anthracis*, a non-motile, Gram-positive, endospore-forming, rod-shaped bacillus. The bacterium generally stays in spore form in the soil and can survive for decades. It is pathogenic, mostly for herbivores, which often get infected while grazing and act as its main host. Hence, the disease in human is usually resultant of contact with anthrax-infected animals or anthrax-contaminated animal products.

Occupational Exposures: The main routes of occupational exposure are:

- dermal contact with contaminated soil, infected animals, infected meat, and animal horns and hides
- inhalation of spores

Workers susceptible to exposure include animal breeders, agricultural workers and hunters, veterinarians and veterinary care workers, butchers and slaughterhouse workers, wool, hair and hide processors, tanners and textile workers, and staff in veterinary and inspection laboratories.

It infection was previously known as '*wool-sorters disease*', because of the association with this work activity. Gastrointestinal exposure to anthrax, though doubtful in occupational settings, may be possible after the consumption of contaminated meat of infected animals. Anthrax spores have been used as biological weapons in a few cases of bioterrorism acts.

Biological Mechanisms and Health Implications: *Bacillus anthracis* spores are infectious and can develop into vegetative bacteria that increase locally after dermal contact or consumption but may also spread causing systemic infection. Inhaled spores are ingested by lung macrophages and carried via the lymphatic system to regional lymph nodes, where they can germinate, multiply, and eventually, invade the bloodstream. Once in the bloodstream, the bacilli release three proteins named lethal factor, oedema factor, and protective antigen. The last one combines with the first two factors allowing cellular entry of these agents causing lethal and oedema toxins, respectively, which are the primary agents of tissue destruction of the host. Invasion of bacilli into the bloodstream can lead to sepsis. Clinical manifestations of anthrax depend on the route of exposure:

- Cutaneous anthrax after skin contact is characterized by a painless itchy skin lesion, together with local oedema, lymphadenopathy, and malaise.
- Pulmonary anthrax subsequent to inhalation is categorized by fever, malaise, non-productive cough, and dyspnoea
- Gastrointestinal anthrax after ingestion is depicted by nausea, loss of appetite, vomiting, and fever, followed by intestinal soreness, haematemesis, and diarrhoea.

Preventive Measures: Impermeable nitrile, vinyl or latex gloves can shield workers from cutaneous exposure to anthrax. Health workers in hospitals, clinics, and medical laboratories, engaged in taking care of patients with suspected exposure to anthrax, must take precautions against the potential for re-aerosolizing any anthrax spores. The safeguards include:

- Housekeeping
- Proper use of gloves
- Protective clothing
- Respiratory protection
- Work practices

Brucellosis: It is a zoonotic disease caused by aerobic coccobacilli of the Brucella genus. It is also known as:

- Bang's disease
- Crimean fever
- Gibraltar fever
- Malta fever
- Mediterranean fever
- Rock or undulant fever

Several species of the microbe infect different mammals which act as its reservoirs for the disease. Its natural reservoirs are sheep, goats, pigs, cattle, dogs, horses, rabbits, rats, voles and red foxes, and marine mammals. Brucella species are Gram-negative, small in size, lack capsules, flagellae, endospores, or native plasmids, and survive in extreme conditions of temperature, pH, and humidity. Even frozen infected materials can be a reservoir of viable, infectious microbes.

Occupational Exposures: Brucellae pose a serious hazard to employees in clinical and veterinary laboratories, agriculture, livestock, dairy industry and slaughterhouses, and meat packers, butchers, and veterinarians. They can reach and infect humans through direct contact or ingestion of products from infected animals. Consumption of infected raw milk remained the most common route of infection before milk treatment. In an occupational setting, the common paths of exposure are breathing in of spores and viable organisms, and dermal contact with infectious material.

Biological Mechanisms and Health Implications: The response to Brucella infection is governed by the virulence, phase, and species of the infecting strain. Exposure to the pathogen produces both cell-mediated and humoral immune responses. The target cells of the infection are the macrophages. Replication of Brucellae takes place in cells of the lymph nodes and subsequent spread through the bloodstream may result in chronic localized infection. The symptoms of disease are flu-like symptoms with:

- Anorexia
- Arthralgia

- Fatigue
- Myalgia
- Pyrexia
- Sweating

The clinical manifestations of the disease occur between two and four weeks after infection. At the beginning, symptoms are non-specific. In some cases, a skin rash can be seen, rarely together with lymphadenopathy and liver and spleen enlargement. The complications observed in chronic forms are:

- Arthritis
- Impairment of Central Nervous System
- Peripheral neuropathy
- Severe endocarditis
- Spondylitis
- Uveitis

Preventive Measures: These involve:

- Pasteurization of milk
- Proper cooking is sufficient to eliminate microbe from food meat
- Vaccination of cattle
- Slaughtering of infected units followed by thorough sanitization or disposal of contaminated pens

Hepatitis Viruses: Viral hepatitis is an infectious disease of liver caused by many viruses:

- Adenovirus
- Cytomegalovirus
- Epstein-Barr virus
- Hepatitis B, C, and A are the major occupational hazards
- Hepatitis E
- Hepatitis G
- Hepato-tropic viruses identified as A, B, C, D, and E

Occupational Exposures: Hepatitis B, C, and D spread through contact with infected human blood and body fluids. Sharp injuries, such as needle-stick accidents, are the most frequent exposure events. The following are more likely to get exposed to these viruses:

- Health workers
- Police and ambulance crews
- Workers in clinical laboratories
- Workers involved in pig breeding and slaughterhouses
- Workers involved in rescue services

In the non-working environment, Hepatitis B and C can be transmitted from carrier individuals mostly by personal relationships:

- Sexual intercourse
- Mother-to-child transmission
- Sharing of personal items

Hepatitis A and E are contracted through the oro-faecal route.

Biological Mechanisms and Health Implications

Hepatitis A: Infection is transferred by contamination of food and water with infected faeces and has an incubation period of two to six weeks. Symptoms include:

- Malaise
- Anorexia
- Nausea
- Vomiting
- Jaundice

Hepatitis B: Infection is transmitted through contact with infected human blood and body fluids with acute and chronic outcomes. Main symptoms include:

- Liver inflammation
- Jaundice
- Flu-like symptoms
- Urticarial rash

The transmission route of Hepatitis C is analogous to Hepatitis B.

Preventive Measures: The preventive measures include:

- Effective organization of work at workplaces mainly handling biological specimens in clinical laboratories, animal breeding farms, and slaughterhouses
- Evading exposure to infected biological material
- Executing engineering control measures in clinical setups
- Minimizing exposure to hepatitis viruses which are transmitted by contact with blood and tissue
- Separation of sewage effluents and tanks
- Undertaking risk assessment and determining exposure

Human Immunodeficiency Virus (HIV): HIV is an RNA retrovirus and its infection usually takes a longer time to progress to symptomatic HIV/AIDS and has a lower death rate than HIV-1 infection.

Occupational Exposures: HIV can be transmitted through:

- Sharing of contaminated needles, syringes, surgical equipment
- Transfusion of contaminated blood
- Transmission from mother to infant during pregnancy, childbirth and breastfeeding
- Unprotected sexual intercourse (vaginal or anal) with an infected person

Occupational exposure occurs if there is a possibility of contact with blood or body fluids at the workplace, for instance through injury caused by blood smeared instruments or inadvertent exposure of the skin, eyes, or mucous membranes. Sex workers are at an increased risk and act as a reservoir for this disease. The route of HIV exposure is:

- Contact through mucous membranes
- Percutaneous injury
- Through non-intact skin (e.g. dermatitis)

The main groups at risk for HIV infection by non-sexual transmission are:

- Health workers
- Laboratory technicians
- Nurses
- Physicians

Other groups at risk of blood or body fluid exposure are:

- Aid agency workers
- Emergency responders
- Fire fighters
- Police officers
- Prison workers
- Waste disposal workers

Biological Mechanisms and Health Implications: The virus targets and attacks the immune system; specifically CD4 cells (T-helper or T4), macrophages, and dendritic cells for CD4 cells play a central role in immune protection.

Preventive Measures: Preventive measures include:

- Infection control precautions like use of gloves, face shields, or other appropriate barriers
- Personal hygiene facilities
- Preventing needle stick injuries which can avoid 90 percent of occupational transmissions of HIV
- Use of safer needle devices and needleless intravenous systems
- Disposing needles and sharps into sharps containers immediately after use

Leptospirosis: Leptospirosis is a zoonotic disease caused by spirochaetes belonging to pathogenic species of the genus Leptospira.

Occupational Exposure: The pathogenic species infect a wide range of animals, which spread the pathogens, colonize the proximal renal tubules, and are shed via urine in the environment. The primary source of leptospires is urine of animals, mainly mice and rats, field rabbits, foxes, horses, and pigs. The infection is transmitted to humans via exposure of mucous membranes or wounded skin to the body fluid of an infected animal or to water or soil contaminated by the urine. The following are exposed to the pathogen at the workplace:

- Agricultural workers
- Banana farmers
- Bathers
- Butchers
- Campers
- Dairy and pig farmers
- Fish handlers
- Forestry workers
- Health workers
- Hunters and trappers
- Laboratory technicians
- Meat packers
- Miners
- Rice and sugarcane fieldworkers
- Rodent control workers
- Sportsmen
- Veterinarians

Biological Mechanisms and Health Implications: Leptospirosis is only zoonotic in origin, and human-to-human transmission has not been documented. Leptospirosis is also known as:

- Seven-day fever
- Cane-Cutter's fever
- Canicola fever
- Fort Bragg fever
- Haemorrhagic fever or infectious jaundice
- Mud fever
- Nanukayami fever
- Pretibial fever
- Rat catcher's yellows
- Rat fever
- Rice field fever
- Spirochaetal jaundice

- Swamp fever
- Swineherd's disease or sewer man's flu

The important source of leptospires is the urinary shedding of organisms from infected animals. Thus, contact with infected urine or urine-contaminated media causes human infection. Leptospires are believed to enter the host through animal and rodent bites, abrasions in healthy skin, mucous membranes or conjunctivae, the placenta during pregnancy, lungs after inhalation, and through ingestion of food and drink contaminated by the urine of an infected animal. Once inside the human or animal, the pathogens reach the bloodstream, ultimately producing leptospiraemia which spread to all organs, although the kidneys and the liver are the most commonly affected.

Preventive Measures: The following preventive measures can help in controlling the pathogen:

- Avoiding smoking, drinking, and eating while handling livestock
- Constant monitoring and testing of livestock
- Creating awareness about the cause and symptoms of the disease, and ways of reducing risk
- Disinfection of living accommodations
- Personal hygiene
- Risk awareness
- Rodent control management
- Vaccination of animals

Tetanus: Tetanus is a life-threatening systemic infection caused by the exotoxins of Clostridium tetani, a Gram-positive, anaerobic, and spore-forming bacillus. Ruminants are natural reservoirs of the spores, which are released with animal droppings, and soil and manure are thus major sources of contamination.

Occupational Exposure: Most workers can be exposed to tetanus infection from open wounds. Occupational groups at risk include:

- Agricultural workers
- Carpenters
- Construction and machinery workers
- Farmers and breeders
- Metalworkers
- Microbiology laboratory workers
- Military personnel
- Miners
- Paper and cardboard manufacturing workers
- Waste workers

Biological Mechanisms and Health Implications: After entering the site of a deep, penetrating wound, the spores find an anaerobic environment, germinate, produce, and secrete two extracellular toxins which cause spasms and rigid paralysis of the muscles.

Preventive Measures: These involve:

- Mass vaccination of the general population
- Using appropriate protective clothing in activities such as agriculture and industrial work
- Providing safety shoes with reinforced, pierce-proof soles and robust gloves to the workers at risk
- Awareness generation

Tuberculosis: Tuberculosis (TB) is a transmissible infectious disease caused by several strains of Mycobacteria. Most human tuberculosis are caused by Mycobacterium tuberculosis.

Reservoirs are mainly humans, diseased cattle, swine, badgers, and other infected mammals.

Occupational Exposure: Tuberculosis can occur in several groups of workers, including:

- Health workers especially during procedures such as bronchoscopy, intubation, and autopsy
- Laboratory technicians and scientific staff working with non-human primates
- Risk of TB is more in oil and gas industries, agriculture, mining, and extractive industries
- Social workers in centres for the displaced and migrants
- Work camps, and trades with a large migrant workforce

Biological Mechanisms and Health Implications: The microbe settles in the lungs and causes scarring of the lung tissue. When macrophages drain from the lung and move to other tissues, they can spread the disease causing extra-pulmonary tuberculosis.

Preventive Measures: These measures include:

- educating, training and counselling people about TB
- evolving and implementing effective policies and protocols
- executing effective work practices among health workers at healthcare facilities
- rapid identification, isolation, diagnostic evaluation, and treatment of infected persons
- screening health workers for TB infection and disease

Engineering controls to prevent the spread and reduce the spreading of infection include:

- air cleaning using air filtration or ultraviolet germicidal irradiation
- direct source control by employing local exhaust ventilation
- eliminating and diluting contaminated air via general ventilation
- monitoring the direction of airflow to prevent contamination of air

6.6.2 Diseases Caused by Chemical Agents

1. **Alcohols, Glycols, or Ketones**

Alcohols are a class of aliphatic hydrocarbon derivatives where one hydroxyl group (-OH) replaces one hydrogen atom. Glycols are a chemical class of aliphatic hydrocarbon derivatives where two hydroxyl groups (-OH) replace two hydrogen atoms on different carbon atoms. Ketones are a chemical class of aliphatic hydrocarbon derivatives where one carbonyl group (>C=O) replaces one internal methylene group (-CH2-).

Occupational Exposures: Lower alcohols, glycols, and ketones are often known as '*oxygenated solvents*' and find technological applications as solvents and as industrial chemical reagents. Occupational exposure to these is possible during their production or using them as initial products or solvents in manufacturing of industrial or consumer products, and managing formulated products containing them. Lower alcohols are used in industry mostly as water-miscible solvents and detergents while specific alcohols are used in organic mixtures. Glycols find numerous different uses in industry and technology. Most of these are used:

- as starting material for production of condensation polymers
- as textile moderating agents and plasticizers
- in brake fluids, greases, mould-release agents, and ink solvents
- in preparations of antifreeze or liquid coolants

Lower ketones are used:

- as starting materials in industrial organic productions
- in formulating inks, resins, varnishes, lacquers, certain glues, surface coatings, paint removers, and automotive care products
- as solvents in cleaning and degreasing

Route of Exposure: Most alcohols, glycols, and ketones can be inhaled as airborne vapours and mists through the respiratory tract, and be more or less absorbed totally. Absorption through the skin is possible since these compounds and complex mixtures of them are often used in formulations and in consumer products. In case of the less volatile compounds, skin absorption is the most probable route. There is a probability of accidental or deliberate ingestion of industrial methanol and ethanol as illegal alcoholic drinks, generally with severe outcomes. Based on their nature and concentration, and duration of exposure, they may cause irritation of the airways. Subsequent to absorption, they are:

- usually bio-transformed in the liver
- enter the pathways of fundamental cell metabolism, such as glycolysis and the Krebs cycle, the biosynthesis of fatty acids, and other biochemical pathways of mineralization

In some cases, their intermediate bio-transformed forms are chemically reactive and can impair biological mechanisms by overloading the biochemical pathways, through inactivation of key enzymes or other specific mechanisms. These compounds are highly reactive electrophiles that can inactivate key enzymes. The un-metabolized fraction of these compounds is excreted in the urine or undergoes very simple biotransformation into conjugates, especially glucuronides and sulphates. During exposure and in the early hours after termination of exposure, the elimination of volatile compounds and some bio-transformed forms occurs in the expired air.

Ethylene glycol is quickly absorbed by the GI tract, while dermal absorption is slow. Because of its very low vapour pressure, exposure by inhalation is generally not linked with toxicity. Acute systemic toxicity from ethylene glycol has been described after ingestion. Ethylene glycol is metabolized in the liver to a variety of compounds of increasing toxicity. The metabolites are accountable for systemic toxicity, since they prevent fundamental biochemical processes, such as:

- Oxidative phosphorylation and cellular respiration
- Glucose and serotonin metabolism
- Protein synthesis
- DNA replication
- Synthesis of ribosomal RNA

The accumulation of organic acid metabolites results in an anion gap metabolic acidosis that affects many cellular functions. Acute systemic ethylene glycol poisoning causes:

- Death in the most severe cases
- Depression of CNS followed by metabolic acidosis
- Pulmonary oedema
- Renal failure with the formation of oxalate crystals

Acetone is absorbed by inhalation and dermal absorption, where it causes mild irritation and enhances absorption of other substances. It is an irritant of upper respiratory tracts at high concentration. Its systemic toxicity is low and lethal doses to be absorbed are questionable. Since it is a natural product of human primary metabolism, most absorbed acetone is mineralized by conversion to acetyl-CoA, while a fraction is eliminated with exhaled air.

Disease Manifestation: Exposure to high concentration of alcohols or ketones (and their vapours) can cause:

- Irritation of eyes and respiratory tract, with rhinitis, laryngitis, and bronchitis
- High exposures to ketone vapours may lead to chemical pneumonitis
- Lung and upper respiratory tract irritation

In case of contact with the eyes, alcohols or ketones or their vapours may produce a local inflammation (conjunctivitis) or corneal ulcers, with altered, reduced, or loss of vision.

2. **Ammonia**

Ammonia (anhydrous) NH_3 is a colourless gas that can be easily liquefied by moderate pressure and cooling to produce a compressed liquid gas. It has a typical pungent odour of decayed urine. NH_3 is usually produced in bulk in industry. It is corrosive for Cu, Al, Zn, and its alloys, natural and vulcanized rubber. NH_3 reacts vigorously with acids, oxidants, and halogens and dissolves easily in water to produce an alkaline solution of NH_4OH.

Occupational Exposure: NH_3 is produced using the Haber process, involving direct reaction of hydrogen usually from methane in natural gas with nitrogen from air, at temperatures higher than 400°C in beds of catalysts containing transition metals. NH_3 is used for manufacturing:

- agricultural fertilizers, nitric acid, synthetic urea, and sodium carbonate
- dyes, pesticides, plastics, explosives, and pharmaceuticals
- fibre monomers, nylon, rubber, and polymer resins
- organic chemicals including acrylonitrile, caprolactam, and diamines
- pulp and paper, food and beverage, textile, leather, and metallurgical processes

It is used as a corrosion inhibitor, and as a neutralizing agent for acidic gases and nitrogen oxides in industrial emissions. Occupational exposure to NH_3 gas occurs mainly from spills or leaks from NH_3 tanks or pipelines. A large amount of gaseous NH_3 is released by the decomposition of biological materials such as sludge from wastewater processing plants, manure, and concentrated animal feed. This can be hazardous in enclosed environments like tanks and pits.

Route of Exposure: NH_3 is a physiological constituent of living matter that undergoes extensive biotransformation to nitrogen-containing molecules and tissues. It is the main product of nitrogen metabolism, which is excreted as urea in the urine. It adds to systemic toxicity of liver and kidney diseases, with neurological impairment, which can cause coma and death. NH_3 dissolves in moisture of skin and mucous membrane to form ammonium hydroxide. It causes saponification of cell membrane lipids, cell disruption, and tissue necrosis. It starts an inflammatory response, which further damages the adjacent tissues. Contact with liquid NH_3 can cause cold injury. The toxic effects are usually limited to tissues in direct contact with NH_3. Exposure to high concentration of liquid or vapour NH_3 causes severe burns in the skin, eyes, upper airways, and GI tract. In the respiratory tract NH_3 can cause laryngeal oedema, pneumonitis, and pulmonary oedema. The permanent effects of NH_3 include visual impairment, and chronic pulmonary disease. Acute diseases caused by NH_3 are:

- Acute chemical pneumonitis and bronchitis
- Chemical burns and corrosions of respiratory tract and eyes
- Conjunctivitis and corneal ulcer
- Irritant-induced occupational asthma
- Laryngitis and pharyngitis
- Pulmonary fibrosis and pulmonary oedema
- Reactive airways dysfunction syndrome
- Respiratory tract irritation
- Rhinitis and sinusitis
- Upper respiratory inflammation

Exposure to NH_3 vapours causes:

- Airway obstruction
- Bronchiolar and alveolar oedema
- Irritation and caustic burns of the respiratory tract, the mucous membranes, and the eyes
- Nasopharyngeal and tracheal burns

Ingestion of ammonium hydroxide, results in erosion of lining of mouth, throat, and stomach.

Clinical Manifestations: Nonspecific symptoms of acute poisoning include:

- Headache
- Loss of sense of smell
- Nausea and vomiting

In severe cases, there may be:

- Agitation
- Airways ulceration and obstruction
- Hypoxia
- Oedema of the mucous membranes
- Pulmonary oedema

Long-term exposures to ammonia vapour can cause:

- Asthma
- Bronchial hyper responsiveness
- Bronchiectasis
- Chronic bronchitis

- Chronic cough
- Chronic irritation of the respiratory tract, mucous membranes, eyes and skin
- Lung fibrosis

Severe cases are accompanied by progressive airway obstruction.

3. **Arsenic or its Compounds**

Occupational Exposure: It occurs in several processes, and those involved in the following viz.:

- Glass-making and optical industry
- Preparation and manufacturing of alloys with other metals (e.g. with lead, copper, zinc)
- Production of microelectronics
- Residual manufacturing using arsenic-containing compounds
- Smelting of sulphide-arsenide ores

Clinical Manifestations: Exposures to arsenic or its compounds can cause:

- Acute toxic encephalopathy
- Arsenical keratosis (warts)
- Chemical bronchitis and pneumonitis
- Chemical pulmonary oedema
- Haematological alterations
- Irritation of mucous and respiratory membranes
- Liver damage
- Lung cancer
- Ulceration of nasal septum
- Plantar hyperkeratosis
- Sensorimotor polyneuropathy
- Skin cancer
- Skin hyperpigmentation
- Upper respiratory inflammation
- Raynaud's syndrome

4. **Asphyxiants like CO, H_2S, HCN or their derivatives**

Carbon Monoxide: It occurs in several processes, and those involved in the following viz.:

- Accidental fires
- Chemical industry
- Coal and fuel furnaces
- Firing of demolition explosives

- Incineration facilities for solid wastes
- Motor vehicle garages
- Poorly ventilated engine rooms
- Tunnel construction works

The main occupations exposed to carbon monoxide are:

- Car mechanics, fire fighters, and garage personnel
- Workers engaged in incineration processes, construction of road tunnel, metallurgical processes, gas, petroleum, and chemical industries

Hydrogen Sulphide: It occurs in several processes, and those involved in the following viz.:

- Anaerobic fermentation of manure for production of biogas
- Extraction of non-ferrous metals
- Farming operations such as stirring of manure
- Industrial uses involved in the hydrodesulphurization of natural gas and crude oil
- Inspection of waste-water canals, sludge pits, burials, and cemeteries
- Leather and petrochemical industry
- Production of sucrose from sugarcane and sugar-beet
- Production of viscose cellulose
- Rotting of natural organic waste
- Sewage water treatment plants
- Textile and leather dyeing

Hydrogen Cyanide: Exposure occurs in the processes, and those involved in industrial synthesis of nitrogen-containing organic compounds.

Sodium Cyanide: Exposure occurs in workers who are exposed both to alkali cyanides.

Potassium Cyanide: Exposure occurs among workers involved in refining platinum, metal colouring, and separating gold, silver, and copper from platinum.

Calcium Cyanide: Exposure occurs among workers involved in using fumigants, manufacturing of cement, stainless steel herbicides, rodenticides, fertilizers, etc.

Clinical Manifestations: Exposures to asphyxiants can cause:

- Acute chemical pneumonitis and bronchitis
- Acute/chronic diseases caused by asphyxiants
- Chemical burns and corrosions of external body surface
- Conjunctivitis and corneal destruction
- Frostbite

- Hypoxic brain injury
- Inflammation of upper respiratory tract
- Irritant contact dermatitis
- Irritant-induced occupational asthma
- Ischaemic heart disease due to CO
- Pulmonary oedema
- Reactive airways dysfunction syndrome (RADS)
- Respiratory tract irritation
- Retinal haemorrhage
- Toxic encephalopathy due to CO, and HCN

5. **Beryllium or its Compounds**

Occupational Exposure: Occupational exposure to beryllium dusts and fumes occurs in:

- Metal extraction
- Refining
- Preparation of beryllium alloys into usable goods by melting, grinding, welding, drilling
- Decommissioning and recycling of beryllium products and waste materials

Clinical Manifestations: Exposures to beryllium or its compounds can cause:

- Acute bronchitis and pneumonitis
- Allergic contact dermatitis
- Berylliosis (acute/chronic)
- Conjunctivitis
- Hepatic granulomas
- Inflammation of upper respiratory tract
- Irritant contact dermatitis
- Lung cancer
- Nodular skin lesions
- Pulmonary oedema
- Ulceration of skin

6. **Cadmium or its Compounds**

Occupational Exposure: It occurs in several processes, and those involved in the following viz.:

- Electroplating
- Heating or welding of cadmium-containing materials
- Inhalation of particles of metal, oxide, and pigment dust
- Manufacturing of battery, plastics, ceramics, paint, and welding operations
- Metal machining

- Production of cadmium alloys
- Smelting, melting, and refining of metals containing cadmium
- Welding, and oxyacetylene cutting of cadmium coated steel and rivets

Clinical Manifestations: Exposures to cadmium or its compounds can cause:

- Acute chemical bronchitis and pneumonitis
- Acute chemical pulmonary oedema
- Anosmia
- Chronic kidney disease
- Fanconi-like syndrome
- *Itai-Itai* disease
- Kidney, lung and prostate cancer
- Nephropathy
- Osteomalacia and osteoporosis
- Pulmonary emphysema
- Reactive airways dysfunction syndrome (RADS)

7. **Chromium or its Compounds**

Occupational Exposure: It occurs in several processes, and those involved in the following, viz.:

- Anti-algal agents
- Antifreeze
- Cement
- Chrome alloy production and chrome electroplating
- Copier servicing
- Glass making
- Leather tanning
- Paints/pigments
- Photoengraving
- Porcelain and ceramics manufacturing
- Production of high-fidelity magnetic audio tapes
- Tattooing
- Manufacturing of textile
- Welding of alloys or steel
- Wood preservatives

Clinical Manifestations: Exposures to chromium or its compounds can cause:

- Acute toxic liver disease and renal failure with tubular necrosis
- Allergic contact dermatitis and allergic disorders of upper airways
- Burns and corrosions of external body surface, eyes, internal organs, respiratory tract
- Chemical bronchitis and pneumonitis

- Chemical pulmonary oedema
- Chrome ulcers, chronic bronchitis, chronic obstructive pulmonary disease (COPD), and chronic rhinitis
- Conjunctivitis and corneal ulcer
- Emphysema
- Irritant contact dermatitis
- Irritant-induced occupational asthma
- Keratitis
- Lung cancer
- Reactive airways dysfunction syndrome
- Ulceration of nose septum
- Upper respiratory tract inflammation

8. **Copper or its Compounds**

Occupational Exposure: Occupational exposure to copper and its compounds can occur in several activities including:

- Alloying
- Copper ore mining, extraction
- Decommissioning and recycling
- Machining
- Soldering
- Synthesis and use of copper compounds
- Thermal and electrochemical metallurgy and refining
- Industries manufacturing/using cupric oxide, cupric hydroxide, copper chromates, copper phthalocyanine

Clinical Manifestations: Exposures to copper or its compounds can cause:

- Allergic contact dermatitis
- Chronic pulmonary fibrosis
- Contact urticaria
- Irritant contact dermatitis
- Metal fume fever
- Respiratory tract irritation and upper respiratory inflammation
- Ulceration of nasal septum

9. **Fluorine or its Compounds**

Occupational Exposure: It is more common among those who are involved in handling of:

- Fluorspar
- Cryolite
- Fluorapatite

- Elemental fluorine and hydrofluoric acid
- Boron trifluoride
- Nitrogen trifluoride
- Carbonyl fluoride
- Oxygen difluoride
- Perchloryl fluoride
- Phosphorus pentafluoride
- Sulphur tetrafluoride
- Chloro-fluoro hydrocarbons

Clinical Manifestations: Exposures to fluoride or its compounds can cause:

- Irritation of mucous membrane
- Upper respiratory inflammation, acute chemical pneumonitis, acute chemical pulmonary oedema, reactive airways dysfunction syndrome (RADS), occupational asthma, chronic obstructive pulmonary disease (COPD)
- Polymer fume fever
- Acute irritant contact dermatitis
- Burns and corrosions of external body surface, eye and adnexa, respiratory tract, internal organs
- Conjunctivitis and corneal ulcer
- Skeletal and dental fluorosis

10. **Latex or Latex-containing Products**

Occupational Exposure: Occupational exposure is common among workers employed in rubber production plants, manufacturing of latex-containing objects, via inhalation of airborne rubber dust and dermal contact. Occupational exposure is common among diverse classes of workers using gloves as personal protective equipment, mainly:

- Healthcare professionals
- Employees of chemical and biological laboratories
- Workers involved in food and catering industry, personal care and hygiene, aestheticians, industrial and household cleaning
- Those working in chemical industry, industrial manufacturing, painting and covering, pesticide application, and public health
- Those involved in farming and livestock rearing

Clinical Manifestations: Exposures to latex or latex-containing compounds can cause:

- Allergic anaphylaxis
- Irritant contact dermatitis
- Allergic conjunctivitis, allergic contact dermatitis, and allergic rhinitis

- Contact urticaria
- Occupational asthma

11. **Lead or its Compounds**

Occupational Exposure: Occupational exposure can occur in:

- Installation and maintenance of structures painted with lead
- Lead pipes, plumbing fittings, and lead linings in tanks
- Mining, smelting, refining, production of metallic lead, alloys, and lead compounds
- Plastics industry
- Production of lead
- Recycling and disposal of lead material and products
- Rubber industry
- Secondary use in the chemical industry
- Shipbuilding and construction industry

Clinical Manifestations: Exposures to lead or its compounds can cause:

- Acute lead nephropathy, cerebral oedema, and acute toxic encephalopathy (organic and inorganic)
- Burn of eye and adnexa, mouth, pharynx and oesophagus, respiratory tract
- Reactive airways dysfunction syndrome (RADS), upper respiratory tract inflammation, irritant-induced occupational asthma, chemical bronchitis and pneumonitis, pulmonary oedema
- Chronic progressive renal failure
- Fanconi-like syndrome
- Gastrointestinal toxicity
- Hypertension
- Male and female infertility
- Irritant contact dermatitis
- Mucous membrane irritation

12. **Manganese or its Compounds**

Occupational Exposure: The main activities involving exposure to manganese are:

- Mining and preliminary treatment of ore
- Manganese refining and making of iron and steel
- Manufacturing of manganese steels

Clinical Manifestations: Exposures to manganese or its compounds can cause:

- Allergic contact dermatitis
- Bronchitis and pneumonitis

- Burns and corrosion of external body surface, eye and adnexa, mouth, pharynx and oesophagus, and respiratory tract
- Irritant contact dermatitis
- Manganism
- Metal fume fever
- Mucous membrane irritation
- Acute/chronic toxic encephalopathy

13. **Mercury or its Compounds**

Occupational Exposure: It occurs in several processes, and those involved in the following viz.:

- Artisan mining industry
- Chemical industry
- Fluorescent lamps, and electric batteries
- Maintenance, repair, and disposal of medical instruments
- Production of sodium hydroxide
- Production of vinyl acetate from acetylene
- Residual manufacturing

Clinical Manifestations: Exposures to mercury or its compounds can cause:

- Acute chemical bronchiolitis and pneumonitis
- Acute conjunctivitis
- Allergic contact dermatitis
- Chemical pulmonary oedema
- Chronic gingivitis
- Chronic kidney dysfunction
- Chronic renal failure
- Disturbances of taste and smell
- Gastrointestinal toxicity
- Irritant contact dermatitis
- Mercury pigmentation
- Toxic encephalopathy
- Toxic nephropathy
- Toxic polyneuropathy
- Upper respiratory inflammation

14. **Mineral Acids**

Occupational Exposure: Occupational exposure is common among those dealing with:

- Acid treatment of metals
- Cleaning agents prior to welding, plating, or painting

- Dye-stuffs
- Manufacturing of isopropanol, synthetic ethanol, sulphuric acid, nitric acid, phosphate fertilizers, soaps and detergent, lead batteries, copper smelting, pickling, etc.
- Metal and wood-working, textile
- Petroleum and photography

Clinical Manifestations: Exposures to mineral acids can cause:

- Mucous membrane irritation
- Acute chemical pneumonitis and bronchitis, upper respiratory inflammation, pulmonary oedema, reactive airways dysfunction syndrome (RADS), irritant-induced acute occupational asthma, chronic obstructive pulmonary disease (COPD)
- Burns and corrosions of eye and adnexa, gastrointestinal tract, external body surface
- Conjunctivitis, blepharoconjunctivitis, keratoconjunctivitis, corneal ulcer
- Acute irritant contact dermatitis
- Acute toxic renal and liver failure
- Chronic skin and mucous membrane irritation
- Erosion of teeth
- Ulceration of nasal septum
- Larynx cancer

15. **Nickel or its Compounds**

Occupational Exposure: Occupational exposure to nickel occurs in:

- Nickel-producing industries (e.g. mining, milling, smelting, and refining)
- Nickel-using industries and operations (e.g. alloy and stainless steel manufacture; electro-plating and electroextraction; welding, grinding, and cutting)
- Industries manufacturing nickel-cadmium batteries, coins, and kitchen utensils
- Recycling operations

Exposure routes in the occupational setting are mainly inhalation and skin contact, while exposure through ingestion rarely occurs.

Clinical Manifestations: Exposures to nickel or its compounds can cause:

- Nickel tetracarbonyl poisoning
- Sensitizer-induced occupational asthma, chemical pneumonitis, pulmonary oedema
- Allergic contact dermatitis
- Chronic rhinitis and chronic sinusitis
- Anosmia

- Ulceration in nose, nasal cavity cancer, paranasal sinuses cancer
- Lung cancer

16. **Organic Solvents**

Occupational Exposure: Workers involved in the following industries are exposed to organic solvents:

- Dry cleaning
- Footwear production
- Industrial painting, floor laying, and lacquering
- Cleaning and degreasing and paint removal
- Industrial printing
- Laboratory and cleaning work
- Maintenance cleaning and repairing of vehicles and machines
- Manufacturing of rubber and plastics
- Pesticides and toiletries
- Production and lamination of reinforced plastic
- Production of paints, lacquers, adhesives, and printing inks

Clinical Manifestations: Exposures to the following organic solvents can cause:

17. **Oxides of Nitrogen**

Occupational Exposure: Workers involved in the following activities are exposed to nitrogen oxides from:

- Arc welding
- Dynamite blasting
- Electroplating
- Engraving
- Factory workers in kilns, furnaces, due to burning of coal, oil, or natural gas
- Manufacturing of civil explosives, rocket fuels, and military ordnance
- Motor mechanics due to exhaust of motor vehicles
- Nitration of organic compounds
- Synthesis of fine chemicals

Clinical Manifestations: Exposures to oxides of nitrogen can cause:

- Irritation of mucous membrane
- Bronchitis and pneumonitis, pulmonary oedema, upper respiratory inflammation, Reactive airways dysfunction syndrome (RADS), irritant-induced acute occupational asthma, chronic obstructive pulmonary disease (COPD)
- Acute irritant contact dermatitis
- Burns and corrosions of external body surface, eye and adnexa

- Conjunctivitis, corneal ulcer, blindness
- Silo fillers' disease
- Methaemoglobinaemia
- Acute effects on CNS
- B_{12} deficiency after exposure to nitrous oxide

18. **Pesticides**

Occupational Exposure: The following workers are engaged in handling of pesticides:

- Workers engaged in the production of commercial pesticides
- Applicators of pesticides in farming and in management of public health issues
- Agricultural workers entering cultivated fields treated with pesticides
- Industrial workers using material or products treated with pesticides
- Non-industrial workers in enclosed spaces treated with pesticides

Clinical Manifestations: Exposures to pesticides can cause:

- Acute pesticide poisoning from chloro-phenoxy herbicides, pentachlorophenol, etc.
- Allergic and irritant contact dermatitis
- Anticoagulation syndrome
- Burns and corrosions of external body surface, respiratory tract, eye and adnexa, mouth and pharynx, oesophagus, and stomach
- Conjunctivitis and corneal ulcer
- Irritant-induced acute occupational asthma, pneumonitis, and acute chemical bronchitis, pulmonary oedema, reactive airways dysfunction syndrome (RADS), upper respiratory inflammation
- Organophosphate-induced delayed neuropathy (OPIDN), acute neurologic effects caused by organochlorinated compounds

19. **Pharmaceutical Agents**

Occupational Exposure: The following are exposed to pharmaceutical agents:

- Chemical workers in pharmaceutical production plants
- Farmers and farm workers
- Health and veterinary workers
- Nurses, pharmacy technicians, surgeons, and medical doctors

Clinical Manifestations: Exposures to pharmaceutical agents can cause:

- Accidental poisoning after exposure to tranquilizers, antidepressants, and anaesthetic gases

- Allergic and irritant contact dermatitis
- Antibiotics resistant bacterial infections
- Carcinogenic effects of antineoplastic drugs
- Congenital malformation syndrome
- Contact urticaria
- Liver failure
- Menstrual disorders and infertility
- Opportunistic/fungal skin and nail infections
- Prolonged bleeding time, coagulation, or prothrombin timing
- Respiratory tract irritation, irritant, and sensitizer-induced occupational asthma
- Vaginitis candidiasis
- Vitamin B deficiency

20. **Phosgene**

Occupational Exposure: Exposure to phosgene can occur while using:

- Cooling fluids in refrigeration systems
- Solvents for metal cleaning and degreasing
- Combustion or high-temperature thermal degradation of chlorinated thermoplastic polymers in industrial
- Production of monomers for polyurethane plastics
- Manufacturing of polycarbonate polymers
- Synthesis of organic intermediates for pharmaceuticals, pesticides, and dyes
- Use of chlorinated fluids as fire extinguishers

Clinical Manifestations: Exposures to phosgene can cause:

- Chemical burns and corrosions of external body surface, eyes, and adnexa
- Conjunctivitis, corneal ulcer, and blurred vision
- Frostbite
- Irritant contact dermatitis
- Respiratory tract irritation, acute chemical pneumonitis and bronchitis, pulmonary oedema, upper respiratory inflammation, reactive airways dysfunction syndrome (RADS), irritant-induced occupational asthma

21. **Sulphur Oxides**

Occupational Exposure: Occupational exposure to sulphur oxides occurs during:

- Burning coal and oil
- Chemical processes of sulphonation of organic acids, vulcanization of rubber
- Food preservation

- Manufacturing of sulphuric acid and oleum in a chemical industry
- Post-combustion treatment of gaseous effluents
- Refrigeration in industrial cooling units

Clinical Manifestations: Exposures to sulphur oxides can cause:

- Acute chemical pneumonitis and bronchitis, chronic obstructive pulmonary disease (COPD), chronic bronchiolitis obliterans, emphysema, pulmonary fibrosis, irritant-induced acute occupational asthma, pulmonary oedema, reactive airways dysfunction syndrome (RADS), upper respiratory inflammation
- Burns and corrosion of respiratory tract, external body surface, eye and adnexa, and other internal organs
- Chronic skin and mucous membrane irritation, acute irritant contact dermatitis
- Conjunctivitis, corneal ulcer, kerato-conjunctivitis
- Darkroom disease
- Irritation of mucous membranes
- Ulceration of nasal septum

22. **Tin or its Compounds**

Occupational Exposure: Occupational exposure to tin is possible in:

- Mining, smelting, and refining
- Production of tin alloys including a large number of non-ferrous alloys
- Industrial soldering in building and in the automobile and electrical industries
- Food and beverage canning industries
- Production of window glass, household utensils, and roofing tiles
- Plastics industry, in production of polyvinyl chloride
- Factories manufacturing disinfectants, molluscicides and antifouling agents

Clinical Manifestations: Exposures to tin or its compounds can cause:

- Burns and corrosions of external body surface, eyes and adnexa
- Cerebral oedema, nephropathy, toxic encephalopathy
- Conjunctivitis
- Contact dermatitis
- Gastrointestinal and hepatotoxicity
- Irritation of mucous membrane
- Severe chemical bronchitis and pneumonitis, pulmonary oedema, upper respiratory inflammation
- Stannosis

23. **Zinc or its Compounds**

Occupational Exposure: Occupational exposure to zinc or its compounds can occur in:

- Extraction of zinc ores
- Smelting
- Refining
- Primary metallurgy activities
- Melting and alloying
- Welding
- Metal recycling
- Manufacturing of chemicals, pesticides, pharmaceuticals and cosmetics, batteries, and recycling
- Preparation of supplemented animal feed and feeding operations
- Moulding and casting machine operators, cleaners, caretakers, and technicians within the metals industry are exposed to zinc

Clinical Manifestations: Exposures to zinc or its compounds can cause:

- Allergic and irritant contact dermatitis
- Burn and corrosion of eyes and adnexa
- Irritation of mucous membranes
- Ulceration of nose
- Upper respiratory tract inflammation

6.6.3 Diseases Caused by Physical Agents

- Diseases caused by compressed or decompressed air
- Diseases caused by exposure to extreme temperatures
- Diseases caused by ionizing radiations
- Diseases caused by optical (ultraviolet, visible light, infrared) radiations including laser
- Diseases caused by vibration (disorders of muscles, tendons, bones, joints, peripheral blood vessels, or peripheral nerves)
- Hearing impairment caused by noise

The diseases caused by physical agents are discussed in detail in Chapter 5 of this book.

BIBLIOGRAPHY

(1984) *Manual of Analytical Methods*. Washington, DC: National Institute for Occupational Safety and Health, US Department of Health and Human Services.

(2008) World Health Organization. *Anthrax in humans and animals*. Available at: https://bit.ly/2Bhzjju.

Faulkner, A. E. and Tiwari, T. S. P. (2020) Tetanus - Chapter 16 in Centres for Disease Control and Prevention's Manual for the Surveillance of Vaccine-Preventable Diseases. Available at: https://bit.ly/38Shtnr.

Hernberg, S. (1992) *Introduction to Occupational Epidemiology*. Philadelphia: Lewis Publishers.

Kasper, D. *et al.* (2012) *Harrison's Principles of Internal Medicine*. New York, NY: McGraw-Hill,

Kraut, J. A. and Kurtz, I. (2008) Toxic alcohol ingestions: clinical features, diagnosis, and management. *Clinical Journal of the American Society of Nephrology* 3(1):208–225.

Lanigan S. (2000) Final report on the safety assessment of Methyl Alcohol. *International Journal of Toxicology* 20:57–85.

Lanigan S. (2001) Final report on the safety assessment of Methyl Alcohol. *International Journal of Toxicology* 20:57–85.

Levy, B. S. and Wegman, D. H. (1994) *Occupational Health: Recognizing and Preventing Work-Related Disease*. Boston: Little Brown.

Lewis, P. (1993) *Health Protection from Chemicals in the Workplace*. Chichester: Ellis Horwood Ltd.

Lewis, R. J. (2000) *Rapid Guide to Hazardous Chemicals in the Workplace*. Chichester: Wiley.

Martin, K. and Bastock, T. W. (1994) *Waste Minimisation: A Chemist's Approach*. London: Royal Society of Chemistry.

Martin, W., Lippitt, J. M. and Prothero, T. G. (1992) *Hazardous Waste Handbook for Health and Safety*. Oxford: Butterworth Heinemann.

McConnell, R. L. and Abel, D. C. (1998) *Environmental Issues: Measuring, Analysing and Evaluating*. New York: Prentice Hall.

Palmer, K. N. (1973) *Dust Explosions and Fires*. London: Chapman and Hall.

Parkes, W. R. (1994) *Occupational Lung Disorders*. Oxford: Butterworth-Heinemann.

Paul, J. and Pradier, C. (1994) *Carbon Dioxide Chemistry: Environmental Issues*. London: Royal Society of Chemistry.

Rosenstock, L. and Cullen, M. R. (1994) *Textbook of Clinical Occupational and Environmental Medicine*. Philadelphia: Saunders.

Schieler, L. and Pauze, D. (1976) *Hazardous Materials*. Wokingham: Van Nostrand Reinhold.

Seifert, S. A., Von Essen, S., Jacobitz, K., Crouch, R. and Lintner, C. P. (2003) Organic dust toxic syndrome: A review. *J Toxicol Clin Toxicol.* 41(2):185–193.

T'So, P. O. and Di Paulo, J. A. (1974) *Chemical Carcinogenesis*. New York: Marcel Dekker.

Vyas, S., Kaur, N., Sharma, N., *et al.* (2009) Methanol Poisoning. *Neurology India* 57(6):835–836.

Wallace, I. G. (1994) *Developing Effective Safety Systems*. Rugby: Institution of Chemical Engineers.

Warren, P. J. (1985) *Dangerous Chemicals, Emergency Spillage Guide*. Walters Samson (UK): New Malden, Surrey.

Wentz. C. A. (1999) *Safety, Health and Environmental Protection*. McGraw-Hill Publishing Company.

Whiston, J. (1991) *Safety in Chemical Production*. Oxford: Blackwell Science.

Young, J. A. (1991) *Improving Safety in the Chemical Laboratory: A Practical Guide*. Chichester: Wiley.

7 Workplace Safety and Health Management

"Safety brings first aid to the uninjured"

—F.S. Hughes

FACT FILE

- Every day, an average of 6,000 people die because of work-related accidents or diseases, adding more than 2.2 million work-related deaths a year. Of these, about 350,000 deaths are from workplace accidents and more than 1.7 million are from work-related diseases
- Additionally, commuting accidents increase the burden with another 158,000 fatal accidents.
- Annually, workers suffer almost 270 million occupational accidents that lead to absence from work for three days or more, and fall victim to some 160 million incidents of work-related disease
- Roughly 4 percent of the world's gross domestic product is lost with the cost of injury, death, and disease through absence from work, treatment of disease, infirmity, and survivor benefits
- Hazardous substances kill about 438,000 workers yearly, and 10 percent of all skin cancers are attributable to workplace exposure to hazardous substances
- Yearly, asbestos alone claims about 100,000 deaths and the figure is increasing
- *Silicosis* – a fatal lung disease caused by exposure to silica dust – still disturbs tens of millions of workers across the globe
- Every year there are at least 60,000 fatal accidents on construction sites around the world. This is one fatal accident every ten minutes
- One in every six fatal accidents at work occurs on a construction site
- In industrialized nations, as many as 25 percent to 40 percent of work-related deaths occur on construction sites, even though the sector hires only 6 percent to 10 percent of the workforce
- In some nations, it is assessed that 30 percent of construction workers suffer from back pains or other musculoskeletal disorders
- The risks a worker faces are governed by their industry, demographics, and other factors
- Improving communication and safety training are the most effective methods to make safety a topmost precedence

DOI: 10.1201/9781003464785-7

- Mental health is the second most important priority at work, with 77 percent of employees saying it is very important to them

7.1 INTRODUCTION

Occupation is an indispensable human activity for which a person spends a considerable part of life for it is stimulating and rewarding but at the same time affects the physical and mental well-being of a person. Health or well-being is not merely the absence of disease but a state of complete physical, mental, social, and spiritual well-being. The World Health Organization defines occupational health as:

> 'the promotion and maintenance of the highest degree of physical, mental, and social well-being of workers in all occupations'

The Joint International Labor Organization Committee on Occupational Health, 1950 defined occupational health as:

> "the highest degree of physical, mental and social well-being of workers in all occupations"

The Joint ILO/WHO Committee in 1950 suggested:

- promotion and maintenance of the highest degree of physical, mental, and social well-being of workers in all occupations;
- prevention from health issues caused by working conditions;
- protection of workers in their occupation from risks of the causes adverse to health;
- placing and maintenance of workers in an occupational environment adapted to their physiological and psychological capabilities

Occupational health is a two-way relationship between work and health and is related to the effects of working conditions and/or environment on the health of workers and influences the ability to perform tasks at the workplace. The maxim, '*Prevention is better than cure*' suggests that work and working conditions do not affect the health of people. The Joint ILO/WHO Committee in 1995 defined the objectives of occupational health as:

- the maintenance and promotion of workers' health and working capacity
- the enhancement of the working environment and work to make it conducive to safety and health
- development of work organization and working culture in a way that supports health and safety at work and thus encourages a positive social climate and smooth operation
- Development of working cultures in a direction, which supports health and safety at work (Health Education) to:
    - prevent occupational hazards/diseases

- achieve maximum human efficiency and machine efficiency
- reduce sick absenteeism

The scope of occupational health practices is confined to:

- prevention of occupational illness and occupational injuries
- promotion of workers' well-being
- decreasing workplace hazards
- restoration of workers' health

7.1.1 Elements of Quality Safety and Health Management

Safety and health rules are common; however, how much action is required will depend on:

- Organization's size
- Hazards presented by the activities at the workplace
- Physical characteristics of the organization
- Products or services manufactured/offered
- Suitability and proficiency of its existing provisions

The success of any organization depends on safety and health management. While the quality management of products/services and environmental fortification mainly protect physical phenomena, safety and health management at the workplace involve caring for and supervising people and evolving a safety culture between employers and employees. Quality management systems encourage constant improvement in all facets of an organization's activities. They are established on a continuous process of:

- classifying the key processes;
- fixing the performance indicators;
- evaluating accomplishment against performance indicators;
- taking remedial measures;
- identifying chances for up-gradation

Success in quality management requires the development of a supportive executive culture. Quality management systems lay emphasis on the significance of the active involvement of all employees in ensuring quality. Organizations that effectively consider safety and health always have a positive culture and active safety programmes. Effective organizations can establish and maintain a supportive culture. Practical methods of planning, constructing, functioning, and sustaining suitable systems are required for the purpose. Elements of quality safety and health management are (Figure 7.1):

A. **Policy and Commitment:** The organization must prepare an occupational safety and health policy programme as part of the Safety Statement.

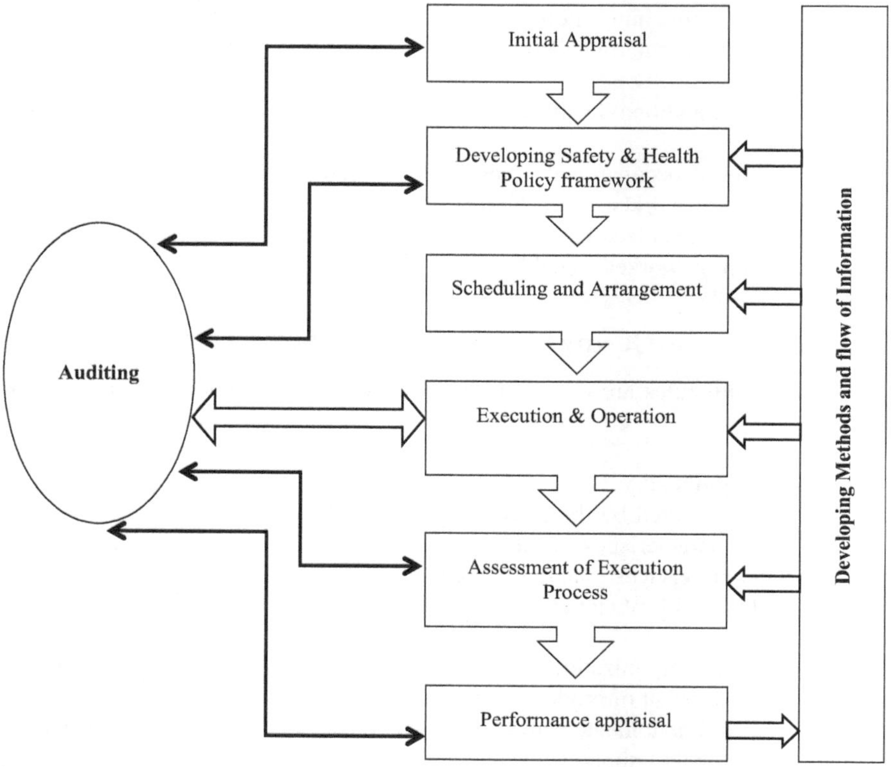

FIGURE 7.1 Key components of a safety and health management system and feedback loop to improve the execution process.

Operational safety and health policies must set a perfect direction for the organization to follow, which must be based on the principle of perceptible commitment to constant improvement. This requires working on cost-effective approaches to preserve and develop human and physical resources that can reduce financial damages and accountabilities. In a broader perspective, stakeholders' anticipations, whether they are shareholders, employees or their senates, customers, or society in general, can be met.

B. **Planning:** The organization must formulate a plan to fulfil its safety and health policy planned in the Safety Statement. An operational management structure and schedule must be evolved for the effective delivery of the policy. Safety and health objectives and targets must be set for all managers and employees.
C. **Execution and Operation:** For effective execution, the organization must evolve the capabilities and support mechanisms required to realize the aims and goals of the safety and health policy. The staff must be inspired and endowed to work carefully and safeguard their long-term health, not

merely to avoid accidents. The arrangement is shown in Figure 7.1. It is ensured by:

- Effective involvement of staff through suitable consultation
- Effective communication and backup of proficiency which permits all employees and their representatives to make an accountable and well-versed contribution to the safety and health endeavour

There must be a strategic and methodical approach for executing the safety and health policy through an operational safety and health management system. The aim must be to curtail risks. Risk assessment methods must be employed to fix priorities and objectives for reducing hazards and risks. Wherever conceivable, hazards must be eradicated through selection and scheming of conveniences, equipment, and procedures. If risks cannot be eradicated, they must be minimalized by using physical controls and safe working systems. Key performance indicators must be indicated for measuring accomplishment. Specific actions to encourage a positive safety and health culture must be categorized. There must be a shared common understanding of the organization's vision, values, and beliefs. The perceptible and dynamic leadership of seniors promotes a positive safety and health culture.

D. **Measuring Performance:** The organization must assess, supervise, and estimate its safety and health operation. Performance can be assessed against established standards to reveal when and where perfection is required. Dynamic self-monitoring shows how efficiently the health and safety management system is working. The objectives of active and reactive monitoring are to:
   - define the instant reasons for poor performance
   - identify any essential reasons and repercussions for design and operation of the safety and health management system
   - monitor long-term objectives

E. **Auditing and Reviewing Performance:** The organization must regularly develop, review, and enrich its safety and health management system so that its overall safety and health performance progresses continuously. There must be an organized review of performance based on data from supervising and from autonomous audits of the entire safety and health management system. There must be a strong commitment to constant improvement including the framing of policies, and the development of risk control systems and techniques. Performance must be assessed by:
   - internal reference to key performance indicators;
   - external assessment based on the show of business contenders

Future challenges for occupational health discipline:

- Ageing working populations;
- Health hazards linked with new biotechnologies;
- New chemical substances and physical energies;
- Occupational health problems linked to new information technologies and automation;
- Occurrence of new occupational diseases of diverse origins;

- Problems of vulnerable and underprivileged groups, including migrants and the jobless;
- Problems related to the growing movement of worker populations; and
- Transfer of hazardous technologies

7.2 EMPLOYERS' RESPONSIBILITIES

It is the legal responsibility of business owners and employers to look into the issues concerning the occupational safety and health of their employees and any visitors to their premises such as customers, suppliers, and the general public. Each country has evolved laws, rules, and regulations to deal with particular hazards depending upon its industrial setup and other requirements. Business owners and employers have engaged a Health and Safety Executive, who is responsible for enforcing health and safety in the workplace. Thus, an employer has a '*duty of care*' to ensure, as much as possible, the health, safety, and welfare of the employee at the workplace. The responsibilities of the employer can be discussed under the following headings:

7.2.1 Risk Assessment

Risk assessment to spot possible health and safety hazards is the initial step in this direction, which requires the engagement of a 'competent person' with health and safety responsibilities. The risk assessment process depends on number of employees, nature of work, and workplace environment; for instance, if an employer engages five or more people, there must also be:

- an official record of the findings of risk assessment
- a formal health and safety policy dealing with the health and safety of an employee

7.2.2 Employers' Accountabilities

All employers, whatever the number of employees, must:

- avoid health risks
- comply with standards, rules, and regulations issued under the government
- confirm that safe working practices are set up and followed
- confirm that the raw material is handled, stockpiled, and used carefully
- confirm that ventilation, temperature, lighting, toilet, washing, and rest facilities all meet health, safety, and well-being standards
- deliver health administration as required
- ensure that machinery is safe to use
- ensure that the proper warning signals are delivered and checked regularly
- examine that the proper equipment is provided, used suitably, and maintained frequently

- make the employees aware of the potential hazards due to work they are involved in – chemicals and raw material used by the firm – and give proper information, guidelines, training, and management as desirable
- make the place of work safe
- prepare emergency strategies
- prevent or control exposure to substances that may harm the health
- prevent potentially hazardous work including manual handling of chemicals, machinery, and equipment
- provide a workplace free from serious identified hazards
- provide access to employee's medical and exposure records to employees or authorized representatives
- provide protective clothing or equipment free of charge
- provide regular medical check-ups and training/counselling as per the standards evolved
- provide safety training in an understandable language and vocabulary for workers/employees
- provide sufficient first aid facilities
- regularly examine the workplace conditions to confirm and comply with appropriate standards evolved by the government/competent body
- regularly update operating procedures and intimate the same to the employees so that they can adhere to the same
- report accidents, injuries, diseases, and hazardous incidences either to the Health and Safety Executive or the local authority, depending on the nature of the same
- take safety measures against the risks caused by inflammable or explosive vulnerabilities, electrical equipment, noise, and radiation
- use colour codes, placards, stickers, or symbols to caution employees of potential hazards

7.2.3 Steps for Making Workplace Safe

In order to provide a safe and healthy workplace, it is important that the employer ensures that:

- raw material is stored safely and cannot cause any harm or injuries to workers
- suitable washing facilities and clean drinking water are provided
- surfaces, pathways, staircases, elevators, and thoroughfares are safe to use
- temperature is at a comfortable level
- there are suitable changing room/resting/dining areas/suitable facilities for pregnant women and nursing mothers
- there is a proper arrangement to protect workers from falling from height
- workplace is clean and well-ventilated, with fresh air
- windows, doors, and gates can be opened whenever required
- working area is big enough to allow easy movement
- working area/premises is properly lighted so that employees can work and move about safely

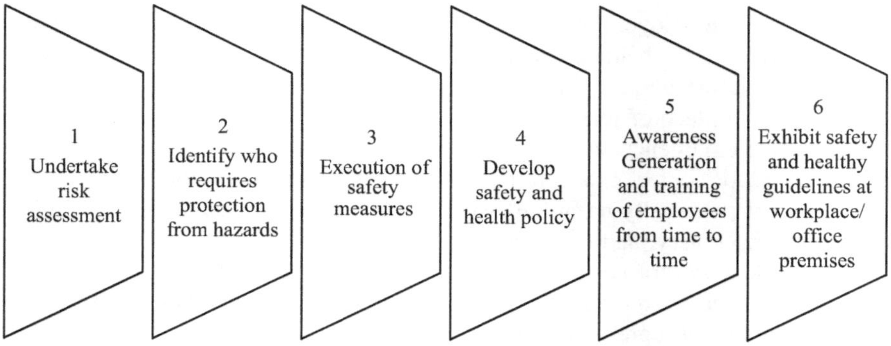

FIGURE 7.2 Steps for making the workplace safe.

- workplace and equipment are clean and are in proper working condition
- workstations are suitable for the employees and the work

Figure 7.2 summarizes the steps involved for making the workplace safe.

7.2.4 Reporting (Injuries, Diseases, and Incidences)

It is the legal obligation of the employer to report the following at the workplace to relevant authorities:

- hazardous incidences
- major injuries
- occupational deaths
- occupational diseases

Reporting Accidents: It is the duty of the employer to report injuries, near slips, fires, or explosions that occurred due to work on or near the electrical systems, incidents arising from leisure and other non-work activities close to the electrical plant, or due to equipment failure.

Conveyance of Explosives: The transport of explosives is covered as per the directives of the state or central government. All employers/companies and individuals must ensure that they are fully informed of the correct way/route of transporting explosives which must comply with the safety standards and lessen the risk of incident.

7.2.5 Record Keeping

Employers are required to keep records on all employees, which help them make decisions about pay hikes, elevations, and sackings. The details they are required to keep include:

- Personal details and contacts/telephone number of family in case of emergency
- Job application form or brief bio-data of employee
- Health/fitness record including the incidence of diseases, any deformity, blood group, etc.
- Employee's behaviour record (employee's attendance, punctuality, and work performance)
- Timesheets (employment contract)

7.2.6 Employees' Duties and Rights

Employees have accountabilities towards their employers, even though they work part-time or don't have any written contract with their employers. The main responsibilities of employees are to:

- arrive at work on time
- attend training provided by the employer
- avoid putting themselves or others in danger
- be faithful to the employer and not disclose confidential information
- carry out their duties as mentioned and specified in the employment contract
- comply with official rules and safety instructions
- follow and abide by the instructions provided by the employer
- personally undertake the work they were hired for
- treat customers, co-workers, and the employer with respect
- undertake their work carefully and seriously
- wear protective equipment and uniform provided by the employer

In case the employees don't render their duties properly, the employer can:

- fire employees if involved in serious incidences, such as stealing from the office
- take disciplinary action against employees, by giving a written warning/ suspending
- take employees to court in case of any criminal offence
- undertake a regular assessment of their performance

Rights of Employees: Employees are secured by law, and have the right to:

- holiday pay
- join a trade union
- receive reasonable allowances and salary
- receive an employment contract
- receive at least the minimum wage
- sufficient rest breaks
- work in a safe and healthy environment, free from danger, bullying, or prejudice

7.3 OCCUPATIONAL SAFETY AND HEALTH MANAGEMENT

The organization/employers must evolve a safety statement and health policy that recognizes and incorporates safety and health an integral part of the organization's key performance indicator.

7.3.1 Developing Safety and Health Policy

The safety and health policy must take into account the:

- hazards and risks associated with the organization's work/activities with a commitment to rationally feasible protection measures for its employees and others;
- commitment to comply with relevant safety and health guidelines backed by the legal framework;
- framework for evaluating the key performance indicators by defining the objectives, targets, appraisal, and re-examining mechanism linked with the safety and health of its employees and other stakeholders;
- clearly understood, executed, and maintained policy at all levels;
- management of safety and health as a prime duty of line management; and
- policy document covering employees' safety and health, participation with well-defined suitable resources to execute the policy

Efficient safety and health management requires comprehensive safety and health policies that are effectively executed and any organization keen on achieving high safety and health standards needs to evolve and develop policies that take into account the:

- need for managers to evolve suitable organizational structures and a work culture that supports risk control;
- role safety and health policy can play in improving the performance level of an organization not only by reducing costs and accountability but as an expression of corporate responsibility;
- the requirement to resource and plan policy implementation effectively;
- the need for comprehending injury, ill-health, and loss by thoroughly identifying, classifying, and assessing hazards;
- the need for an organization to be receptive to any internal and external change;
- the need to scrutinize and review performance and learn from experience; and
- the linkage between quality, environment, safety, health, and good management practices

7.3.2 Characteristic Features of Policy Document

Firstly, the safety and health policy must be a part of the safety statement. The characteristic features of a good policy document are that it must:

- address the employees' responsibilities
- be precise and must be in a written format
- contents of the policy must be based on the hazards and risks associated with an organization and must ensure that methodical hazard identification and risk assessment have been undertaken
- define the safety and health responsibilities of each and every one supervising the execution of policy
- include a commitment that safety and health legislation will be complied with
- specify and fix the accountability of those responsible for implementing the policy at different levels
- specify that adequate resources will be provided for critical safety and health issues, such as the design, provision, and maintenance of:
    - any article, plant, equipment, or machinery at the workplace in a safe manner;
    - desirable safety and health information, instruction, training, and supervision;
    - emergency plans and first-aid training;
    - on-going hazard identification and risk assessments, and compliance with the general principles of prevention as defined in the concerned legislation;
    - reporting of accidents and happenings to the concerned authority for investigation and further necessary action;
    - safe entry and exit from the workplace;
    - safe workplace for all employees;
    - safety and health consultation, employee participation in safety programmes;
    - systems of work that are planned, organized, performed, maintained, or revised; and
    - welfare facilities and PPE

The policy document must be reviewed and updated from time to time to prevent adverse effects on the health and safety of employees. It is essential that those involved in keeping safety and health control systems must be aware of their responsibilities. While framing the policy, the standards, codes of practice, guidelines, industry practices, and linked legal framework of the nation must be considered. The policy document must specify the disciplinary actions for non-compliance.

Thus, in general, the policy must incorporate the aforementioned points; however, the provisions, guidelines, and safety measures depend on the risks associated with work in the organization. For instance, organizations dealing with hazardous material must take into consideration the required guidelines/procedures associated with the handling of the hazardous material. Before implementation, the policy must be placed before the executive/governing bodies of the organization, and legal opinion may be sought before implementation to cover the legal issues, if any, that may be of some trouble in the future.

7.3.3 Planning

Planning is one of the essential components required for the implementation of safety and health policies. Adequate control of risks can be accomplished only through collaborative action ensuring the participation of all members of the organization. An effective planning system requires a safety and health management system that:

- controls the risks and complies with safety and health regulations;
- promotes and sustains a positive safety and health culture;
- responds to changing circumstances and demands;
- supports constant improvement in safety and health performance;

To begin with, the organization must:

- access and identify relevant legislation, codes of practice, and guidelines;
- convey relevant information to the employees; and
- monitor legal and other requirements

Safety and health objectives and targets must be based on legal and other requirements. There must be a blueprint to fulfil the safety and health policy, objectives, and targets, which must include the following:

- distinct timeframe for accomplishing the tasks;
- fixing the accountabilities;
- precise performance indicators; and
- well-defined work programmes – the roadmap for achieving each objective

Thus, a strategic plan with the aforementioned features will certainly help the organization meet its legal obligations and make improvements in its performance.

Another thing that is important here is that the safety and health objectives and targets are realistic and achievable and must be clearly defined to meet the requirements of the organization's safety and health policy. Each objective must be aimed and focused on an overall improvement in safety and health performance and it must be accompanied by precise performance indicators. The objectives of the policy must comply with the applicable safety and health legislations of the organization. The objectives must reflect the aim of risk reduction. Quantifiable targets must be approved by all managers accountable for executing the plan.

7.3.4 Performance Indicators

Performance indicators are the basis of planning, measuring, and realizing safety and health goals. In case the organization believes in efficient and effective risk management, it must coordinate its activities to ensure that everyone is clear about what is expected to be achieved. Defining the key performance indicators is essential if policies are to be translated from good intentions into a series of synchronized activities and tasks. Performance indicators must:

- clearly specify how the stakeholders can contribute to an environment free of injuries, ill-health, and loss;
- form the basis for measuring organizational performance;
- identify the competencies, expertise, and training individuals require to fulfil their respective accountabilities

The process involves the following steps:

- preparing strategies to execute the safety and health policy;
- undertake risk assessments in agreement with specific guidelines;
- intermittent supervision of safety and health policy execution;
- examining contractors' competence regarding safety and health performance before signing an MoU or assigning the job;
- holding administrators' routine meetings on safety and health, which may incorporate imparting of training, for instance, first aid after an accident

The execution of the aforementioned tasks involves:

- Defining a clear timeframe for these tasks
- Referring to legal obligations
- Adequate accomplishment of itemized procedures
- Using output standards to specify how individuals can be held responsible for their safety and health accountabilities.

7.3.5 Execution and Operation

Though the accountability of effective execution and operation of policy ultimately rests with the employer, which is generally delegated to executive directors, senior managers, line managers, supervisors, and employees with clearly defined duties and responsibilities of each, the involvement of each and every one working in the organization can surely be beneficial.

A. **Role of Executive Members**

The organizational and reporting structure for executing the aforementioned responsibilities must be shown in an in-house chart depicting the organizational structure. Furthermore, each board executive must accept the accountabilities and has an obligation toward safety and health issues.

Accidents, disabilities, and events are occasional arbitrary events, which are usually resultant of control failure besides multiple causative factors; however, the instant cause may be a human or technical failure, and such events generally occur due to organizational negligence which is the onus of management. In order to execute effective safety and health management systems, the organization must utilize the manpower assets, viz. managers and other employees. Thus, the safety proclamation must talk about the appointment of a senior manager with executive responsibility and authority for the development, execution, periodic review, and evaluation of the safety and health management system. While implementing the policy, the main focus must be on:

- categorizing and allocating resources for safety and health;
- checking whether objectives and targets have been met;
- ensuring that an appropriate organizational structure is in place;
- ensuring that the safety and health policy is successfully implemented;
- establishing clear-cut reporting relationships;
- evolving plans to execute the safety and health policy;
- evolving safety and health strategies for key high risks;
- explaining job descriptions that include safety and health accountabilities;
- employing necessary improvements after carrying out risk assessments;
- offering all stakeholders the necessary safety and health precautions while delivering services;
- reviewing the effectiveness of the safety and health management system;
- setting safety and health objectives/targets for employees;

B. **Individual Responsibilities**

Though managers and supervisors have direct responsibility for the safety and health of employees, the individual employees also have a duty to ensure their own safety which is generally defined in safety and health and must be conveyed to the duty holders. Individual responsibilities must also be defined in the organization's safety statement. Integration of knowledge and experience through commitment, and involvement means that safety and health in fact becomes everyone's concern. The board of directors or other senior management regulatory body must confirm the active participation of workers in refining safety and health by:

- actively encouraging and sustaining worker participation in all phases of safety and health management system;
- ensuring a safety discussion;
- inspiring partnership for prevention, where workers and the safety representative are involved in categorizing hazards and controlling actual problems;
- making workers aware of their safety and health accountabilities;
- enabling beneficial cooperation and consultation on safety and health matters between employer and employee;
- review the safety statement from time to time

To effectively execute the policy, it is important that consultations with stakeholders are organized from time to time for making constant improvements. Regular consultation can help in conveying to each and every one about novel technology, equipment, or chemicals and their effect on working environments. In addition, they can be made aware on:

- outcome of risk assessments on workplace hazards;
- planning and organization of safety and health training
- safety and health information;

C. **Safety and Health Management System**

Procedures for identifying, maintaining, and arranging safety and health records must be established and sustained. Records must be appropriate to the organization and its safety and health management system, and must include:

- Training records
- Safety-health records (results of noise and air quality monitoring certification)
- Audits and reviews

Safety and health records must be:

- in either electronic or written form, readable, and easily understood by those who have to use them;
- recognizable, and traceable to the activity;
- stored and maintained so that they are protected against damage, deterioration, or loss, and are quickly accessible

Their retaining time must be established and recorded, and comply with legal requirements.

D. **Operational Control Workplace Precautions**

To avoid injury and ill-health at the workplace is the ultimate goal of any safety and health management system. Adequate safety measures must be provided and maintained at the workplace to avoid harm to people at risk. Therefore, workplace precautions to match the hazards and risks are required at each stage, which may include provisions such as machine guards, exhaust ventilation, safety instructions, and proper working systems. The operational control workplace precautions involve:

Risk Control: It is the basis which ensures that suitable workplace safeguards are delivered and upheld. At the input stage, the purpose is to reduce hazards and risks. At the process stage, the focus is on having risks linked with the process. At the output stage, risk control must avoid the export of off-site risks. The nature and relative significance of risk control differ according to the nature and hazard profile of the industry and workplace safeguards. Organizations need risk controls suitable to the hazards arising from their activities and sufficient to cover all hazards.

The design, dependability, and intricacy of each risk control method must be proportional to the hazards and risks involved.

Evolving Workplace Precautions: The risk control is essential to comply with the needs and the appropriate statutory provisions of a nation or an organization. There are three steps in instituting workplace precautions:

- identification of potential hazards that could cause harm;
- risk assessment – assessing any risk that may arise from recognized hazards; and
- risk control – deciding the suitable measures to eradicate or control risk

Hazard Identification: It includes a critical appraisal of all activities and take account of potential hazards to employees, others affected by the organization's activities (e.g. visitors, public, and contractors), and those using its products and services. Attention must be given to hazards arising from routine and non-routine operations. To ensure a methodical documentation of hazards, the organization may refer to appropriate safety and health sources of information, such as:

- accident, ill-health, and incident data of the organization itself;
- applicable national and international standards;
- awareness and experience of managers and employees;
- body imposing safety and health guidance/law;
- expert advice and opinion from competent safety and health professionals;
- important industry or trade association guidance;
- information of articles and substances for use at the workplace;
- legislation/safety and health codes, which give information about the basic minimum requirements; and
- safety and health web links of competent authority

There must be a critical evaluation of all routine and non-routine activities. Employees and Safety Representatives can make a valuable contribution in recognizing the hazards. Hazards can be recognized by observation and by linking the situations with the appropriate information. Expert advice may be required to select and apply the most suitable method.

Risk Assessment: There is a general requirement to carry out a written risk assessment under the relevant statutory provisions. It is essentially concerned with assessment of the gravity and probability of harm arising from recognized hazards. Assessing risks to help determine workplace precautions can be qualitative or quantitative. Risk assessors need knowledge of the activities and working practices being undertaken. Again, the acquaintance of employees and Safety Representatives can prove useful. Risk assessment must be carried out by competent and suitably trained people. Professional safety and health advice may be required in some cases, mainly while choosing suitable Quantified Risk Assessment (QRA) techniques and interpreting results. The risk assessments must be repeated as and when required, e.g. on the introduction of new technology, new work procedures, or processes.

Risk Control: After analysis and assessment, the risk assessors can take decisions about workplace precautions. The decisions about risk-control methods must take into account the applicable legal requirements for they establish minimum levels of risk prevention or control. The employers must implement the following hierarchy of risk control measures:

- Eradication or replacement which is an everlasting solution that removes the hazard completely or replaces one that presents a lower risk;
- Engineering controls or safety measures to reduce the risk (including the use of machine guards, isolation or enclosure of hazards, local exhaust ventilation, mechanical handling methods, or protective barriers);
- Administrative controls to reduce or eliminate exposure (by adherence to procedures or instructions, including supervision, permit-to-work systems, and job rotation);
- Personal Protective Equipment (PPE) (suitable training in the use and selection of PPE is an important to control risk)

The regulatory norms for risk assessment are the same as those for safety. But, the nature of health risks can link the work activities and employee ill-health. Health may be permanently damaged before the risk becomes obvious; hence, it is necessary to develop a preventive strategy to identify and control risks before anyone is exposed to them. Health risks due to work activities include various health implications, some of which are listed in Table 7.1.

TABLE 7.1
Potential Health Impacts of Exposure to Workplace Conditions

#	Type of Substance/Workplace Conditions	Potential Health Impact
1.	Irritant substances due to skin contact	Dermatitis
2.	Inhalation of respiratory sensitizers	Triggering immune responses such as asthma
3.	Awkward body postures or repetitive movements	Upper limb disorders, repetitive strain injury, or other musculoskeletal conditions
4.	High noise level	Deafness and conditions like tinnitus
5.	Excessive vibration from hand-held tools	Hand-arm vibration syndrome and circulatory problems
6.	Ionizing and non-ionizing radiation including ultraviolet from the sun's rays	Burns, sickness, or skin cancer
7.	Inhaling air contaminated by microbiological organisms	Infectious diseases ranging from minor sickness to life-threatening conditions
8.	Job stress	Mental or physical illness

Management of health risks needs advice from professional advisers, like technical staff or occupational health hygienists, nurses, and occupational physicians. Taking the following measures can help in reducing the health risks linked with the workplace:

- referring the workforce while designing the workstations;
- communicating with the suppliers of raw material and equipment;
- enclosing machinery to cut down noise or fumes;
- studying the use of less hazardous materials;
- ensuring the training of staff in the safe handling of all substances and materials; and
- well-timed surveillance

An appositely trained occupational health physician must supervise the design and execution of a proper health surveillance system, though, where suitable, it can be done by an aptly qualified person. Although specialist help may be required to control health risks, employers themselves are accountable for managing work activities in such a way that it affects them minimally.

Monitoring and Measuring Performance: The firm's executive board of directors or senior management team must ensure the relevant safety and health risk management issues. It is suggested that the controlling bodies appoint at least one 'safety and health director' who will ensure that safety and health responsibilities are appropriately performed by:

- appointing a senior officer and conferring executive duty for executing safety and health management system;
- being kept informed about any important safety and health failures;
- confirming that safety and health risk management systems are intact and remain operational;
- effective monitoring and reporting on safety and health performance;
- ensuring safety and health management system;
- ensuring the safety statement and health priorities; and
- yearly reviewing the safety and health performance

Thus, processes to monitor, measure, and record safety and health performance on a regular basis must be created, ascertained, and revised intermittently. The organization must measure what it is doing to execute its safety and health policy and assess how efficiently it is controlling risks. Like planning, supervising safety and health performance against scheduled plans and standards must be a line-management duty, for it strengthens management's commitment to safety and health goals and helps to build a positive safety and health culture. Two types of monitoring are required:

- Active systems (for monitoring the design, development, installation, operation of management arrangements, safety systems, and workplace precautions)

- Reactive systems (for monitoring accidents, ill-health, incidents, and other evidence of underprovided safety and health performance)

The monitoring system must include:

- identification of the appropriate data;
- monitoring of the achievement of specific plans;
- setting performance indicators;
- installation of the requisite monitoring equipment;
- assessment of accuracy and reliability of the required monitoring equipment;
- calibration and regular maintenance of equipment;
- analysis of monitoring data collected;
- data evaluation as a part of the safety and health management review;
- standard procedures for reviewing the monitoring of safety and health implications of changes (if any) to work systems

The following methods must be used for active assessment of the safety and health management system:

- systematic inspections of workplace processes, e.g. weekly, monthly, or quarterly reports;
- systematic review of the organization's risk assessments;
- plant or machinery inspections;
- environmental sampling for dusts, chemical fumes, noise, or biological agents; and
- analysis of safety and health management system records

Auditing and Reviewing Performance: Monitoring gives an idea to let the company review its activities and resolve how to improve its performance. Auditing and performance review are the ultimate stages in the safety and health management control cycle. They create a 'feedback loop' that allows an administration to strengthen, uphold, and develop its capability to reduce risks to the fullest extent and to confirm the constant efficacy of its safety and health management system. Audits, by the organization's own staff or outsiders, can complement monitoring activities. Outcomes of performance must be integrated with information from audits to improve the organization's inclusive approach to safety and health management.

The organization must establish and maintain a programme and processes for regular safety and health management system audits to enable a critical assessment of all elements of the safety and health management system. These audits must be carried out in addition to routine monitoring, inspection, and surveillance to ensure the continuous appropriateness, suitability, and efficiency of the safety and health management system. The audit process must ensure that the necessary information is gathered to allow management to effectively carry out evaluation. The firm must establish and maintain audit records consistent with the safety and health management system and these must comply with legal requirements. Organizations should have a feedback to establish whether their safety and health management system is working efficiently. The main information comes from assessing activities and conducting audits of risk-control systems and workplace precautions. Suitable performance indicators must be evolved to identify the accountabilities, timing, and systems involved. Reviews must examine:

- the operation, maintenance, and efficiency of the system; and
- the design, development, and installation of the safety and health management system

The firm must decide the frequency of reviews at each level and evolve reviewing activities corresponding to the measuring and auditing of activities. Key performance indicators for reviewing overall performance must include:

- assessment of the degree of compliance with the safety and health system and legal requirements;
- recognizing the areas where the safety and health system is absent or inadequate;
- valuation of the accomplishment of specific objectives and plans; and
- accident, ill-health, and incident data supported with underlying causes, trends, and common features

Performance indicators need to be consistent with the development of a positive safety and health culture. Organizations may 'benchmark' their performance against other organizations by comparing the accident rates and management practices and techniques. The safety and health indicators of a firm must be compared with others so as to improve the performance. Besides this, arrangements must be made to ensure the continuous improvement of the safety and health management system.

7.4 WORKERS' PARTICIPATION, TRAINING, ORGANIZATIONAL ASPECTS

Adequate arrangements must be in place to ensure that the employees have the necessary skills to safely perform their work, which requires training. The managers and experts effectively dealing with safety and health must be aware of the legal implications of workplace issues. The companies must have good arrangements including:

- staffing and appointment processes that ensure employees have the necessary physical and mental abilities;
- systems to recognize safety and health training needs;
- training appropriate to the size and activity of the firm;
- refresher course to maintain or enhance competence;
- arrangements and resources to provide information, instruction, training, and supporting communications; and
- general health promotion and surveillance schemes

Proper supervision ensures the development and maintenance of capability and is mainly required for those new to a job or undergoing training. The organization must identify its training needs and implement a training programme that takes into account legal requirements on safety and health training. Training records must be retained. Firms should monitor legal developments to ensure persistent compliance with legal procedures, technical developments relevant to risk control, and developments in safety and health management practice. In case the safety and health policy is to be understood and constantly executed, some key facts must be agreed efficiently and must cover:

- the significance and purpose of the policy;
- the vision, values, and beliefs underlying the policy;
- the obligation of senior management to its execution;
- plans, standards, procedures, and systems linked with enactment and evaluation of performance;
- factual information to secure the participation and assurance of employees and their safety representatives;
- remarks and thoughts for enhancement;
- performance reports;
- lessons learned from accidents/incidents

Visible behaviour, written communications, and face-to-face discussions can provide an adequate flow of information throughout the organization. These methods use both formal and informal means. Firms need to pass safety and health information to others including information about the:

- accident or ill-health or letters of compliance to the Health and Safety Authority;
- the safety of articles and substances supplied for use at work; and
- emergency planning

Hence, special arrangements are required for maintaining lines of communication at the time of crises.

7.5 HEALTH PROMOTION, EDUCATION, AND TRAINING

Workplace safety training is as vital as workplace safety itself. It allows the management to ensure a safe and healthy working environment and helps the employees to recognize safety hazards and correct them. It also empowers them to realize best safety practices and opportunities. Safety training is essential for understanding the safety practices related to their jobs; else, a worker will find himself/herself at a higher risk for workplace injury, illness, or death. There are various reasons to conduct training for employees, for it trains them on the basics of health and safety with increased:

- ability to adopt new skills and methods;
- change in scheme and products;

- company image;
- effectiveness in procedures, springing in financial gain;
- employee income;
- employee motivation;
- focus of employees on their tasks;
- job satisfaction and confidence;
- productivity and satisfaction among personnel; and
- risk management

Workplace training inculcates learning and earning money while working. Apprenticeship is a type of workplace training. It is an efficient act of enhancing knowledge and technical skills of an employee for doing a specific job. Training provides the employees the means which help them emerge as safety professional. The aim of workplace safety training is to:

- bring about modification in the attitudes of the employees towards colleagues, manager, and the organization;
- decrease damage or loss to non-human factors like equipment, machinery, and stocks;
- equip employees with the ability to protect themselves against accidental injuries and death;
- make employees use the materials, machines, and equipment efficiently;
- reduce the number of mishaps by offering safety training to the employees;
- supply job-related knowledge and skills to the employees;
- transmit skills among the employees frequently so that they may learn fast;

Education and training are vital tools for updating workers and managers about workplace hazards and controls so that they can work more safely and be more useful. Effective training and education can be provided outside a formal classroom setting. Peer-to-peer training, on-the-job training, and worksite demonstrations can be effective in communicating safety concepts, ensuring understanding of hazards and their controls, and encouraging good work practices. It can be achieved in various steps and involve different actions, which are highlighted in Figure 7.3.

7.5.1 Training Manual on Occupational Safety and Health

It is essential that the training manual/material to be used for imparting the training on Safety and Health issues must impart knowledge and skills to the management committee members, Doctors, Engineers, Paramedics, and Safety supervisors who act as the working force for a safe and healthy work environment. It should enable them to gain up-to-date knowledge on the concepts of occupational safety and health; keep the workplace safe and healthy and carry out suitable and effective measures and practices, and contribute to the consistency of relevant workplace safety information and sustainability of activities at the workplace. The manual must help the learner to:

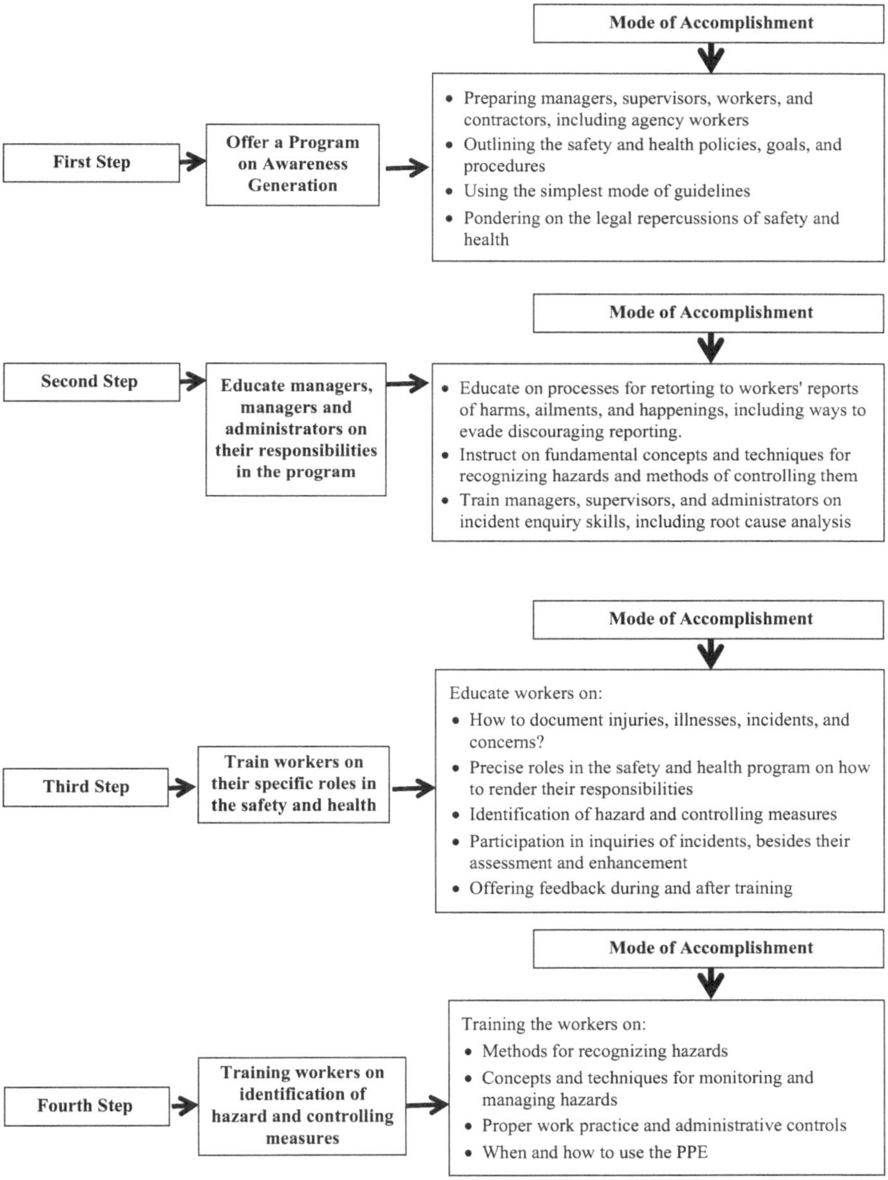

FIGURE 7.3 Steps and approaches of achievement for stimulating health, education, and training.

- discuss the issues pertaining to occupational safety and health;
- explore the way outs for improving workplace health and safety;
- identify workplace health hazards; and
- work out appropriate measures to be undertaken

Safety Management Programme: The significance of a well-planned safety management programme is known to all, but regrettably not executed by everyone. A company's capability to keep its workers safe is governed by its skill to design, execute, and mend the safety management processes and programmes within its enterprise. The top companies in the world prioritize workers' health and safety in a strategic way to make it a shared accountability that enables them to efficiently practice avoidance while preparing them to meritoriously handle any happening that may occur. An effective safety management programme must:

- Reduce the threat of workplace injuries, and fatalities through data-driven dimensions and improvements
- Involve different people in a company to make safety a shared duty
- Be well-arranged to confirm uniform development and performance
- Be practical, protective, and unified with the ethics, morals, values, and standards of the entire organization

The important components of a successful safety management programme:

1. **Ratified Safety Policies:** To outline the organization's safety policies and the importance of safety management are the basic steps of any organization. Safety policies must incorporate judicious operating information for employees to follow all through their working life. These policies must include everything from general operating processes to detailed instructions for dealing with injuries if somebody is injured at the workplace.
2. **Effective and Regular Communication:** It is important that safety policies are often communicated and available to everyone. Intensive and unfailing messages about safety and health can create dedicated, productive, and responsible workers.
3. **Backing for behaviour-based safety:** The safest firms always recognize the significance of inventing and initiating habits around safety and focus on behaviour-based safety – a safety methodology that focuses on refining safety via habit formation. Firms can create good behaviour by developing positive habits while breaking old ones. A framework of 3Rs of Habit Change, viz. **Reminder** (that initiates the behaviour); **Routine** (the behaviour itself) and **Reward** (the benefit from changing behaviour) can help in this regard.
4. **Using both imperative and lagging indicators:** Firms with outstanding safety management systems develop a methodical process to measure what's going on all through the entire safety operation that enables them to quickly understand if something went wrong.
5. **Avant-garde devices and systems:** Firms with low-injury rates provide their workers the cutting-edge tools and systems to keep them prepared and ready to handle whatsoever they need to.
6. **Regular Safety Training and Deliberation:** The safest firms recognize the importance of constant education of their workers, and they highlight

it. The safety training provides managers, employees, and supervisors with:

- Knowledge of proper practices to safely perform their duty;
- Cognizance of how to remove hazards to lessen the risk;
- Speciality when their precise roles require exclusive preparation

These components play important role in reducing incident frequency while refining entire safety. At times, the workers feel bored attending the training sessions; therefore the training sessions must be engaging, fun, and effective for everyone.

7. **Inspired and Driven Workers:** Empowering employees in safety management can help in remarkable outcomes for any organization. Effective safety management programmes and plans constantly encourage proper safety through constant education, steady reinforcement, and continuous improvements.
8. **Sensible Reporting:** It is important that the issues related to safety be reported in time. It must be ensured that the employees realize that safety is the top priority. Employees must feel involved and obliged to report a hazard or potential issue as and when they come across it. Inculcating a sense of responsibility is essential for undertaking safety policies and procedures.

7.5.2 Training Methods and Materials

Learning Objectives: At the end of a session, the participants must:

- have their learning materials;
- understand the aim and structure of the course; and
- have the opportunity to introduce themselves and familiarize themselves with each other

Duration: 30 min

List of Contents

01. Introduction and History of Occupational Health
02. Occupational Safety and Health and Role of Stakeholders
03. Occupational Safety and Health Legislations
04. Occupational Hazards
05. Occupational Diseases
06. Personal Protective Equipment
07. Identification of potential hazards and their health outcome at different workplace
08. Occupational Health and Safety Checklist

Training Method

- Lecture
- Demonstration/display

- Group Discussion and Group Work
- Question and Answer Session
- Fieldwork
- Feedback

Training Schedule

- Orientation
- Fieldwork in the respective area for making observations and collecting data according to the checklist
- Preparation of Report
- Re-orientation
- Feedback and Experience Sharing

The sample of a two-day training programme is shared in Box 7.1.

BOX 7.1 GENALIZED FORMAT OF A TWO-DAY TRAINING PROGRAMME

Day One
Course Content
Session 1: Inaugural Session

- Background Training sessions/defining the learning objectives and brief about the session plan

Session 2: Introduction and History of Occupational Health

- Occupational Safety and Health in Bangladesh

Session 3: OSH Legislations
Session 4: Occupational Hazards
Session 5: Occupational Diseases

Day Two
Session 6: Review
Session 7: Occupational Diseases
Session 8: Personal Protective Equipment
Session 9: Case Studies – hazards and health outcomes at different workplace
Session 10: Hazard Assessment
Session 11: Re-Orientation and Feedback
The re-orientation and feedback session must focus on:

- Re-orientation
- Presentation of Reports and Experience Sharing

- Discussion
- Group Work
- Group Presentation
- Discussion and Feedback

Session 12: Valedictory Session

General Instruction for the Organizer

The organizer involved in imparting the training must:

- prepare the content of the manual and training process before training for acquiring proper knowledge about the subject and effective delivery during the training;
- prepare the training material to be used in the training session like hand-outs, etc. along with multimedia presentation;
- make the learning material available to the participants before each session;
- ensure the attention of every participant and provide a chance to share their experience and opinions to make the training more effective and participatory;
- give equal attention to each participant and treat all participants equally;
- make an effort to attract the attention of each participant;
- be careful that the discussion is always pertinent;
- ensure that the training environment is open and spontaneous;
- mention the content of the session so that the participants can understand the topic;
- conclude each session with key highlights of the topic discussed;
- ensure that the training is conducted confidently

BIBLIOGRAPHY

Aburumman, M., Newnam, S. and Fildes, B. (2019) Evaluating the effectiveness of workplace interventions in improving safety culture: A systematic review. Safety Science 115:376–392.

Allender, S., Colquhoun, D. and Kelley, P. (2011) Competing discourses of workplace health. Journal for the Social Study of Health, Illness and Medicine 10(1):75–93.

Alli, B. (2001) Fundamental Principles of Occupational Health and Safety. Geneva: International Labour Organization.

Bradbury, W. (2019) Three overlooked elements of a successful safety culture. Professional Safety 64(2):22–23.

Christian, M. S., Bradley, J. C., Wallace, J. C. and Burke, M. J. (2009) Workplace safety: A meta-analysis of the roles of person and situation factors. Journal of Applied Psychology 94(5):1103–1127.

CIS. (1998) Chemical Safety: Training Modules International Occupational Safety and Health Information Centre. Minsk, Belarus: Commonwealth of Independent State.

Claxton, G., Hosie, P. and Sharma, P. (2022) Toward an effective occupational health and safety culture: A multiple stakeholder perspective. Journal of Safety Research 82:57–67.

Cunningham, T. R., Tinc, P. J., Guerin, R. J. and Schulte P. A. (2020) Translation research in occupational health and safety settings: Common ground and future directions. Journal of Safety Research 74:161.

Dawson, P. and Zanko, M. (2011) Occupational health and safety management in organizations: a review. International Journal of Management Reviews 14(3):328–344.

Driscoll, T., *et al.* (2005) Review of estimates of the global burden of injury and illness due to occupational exposures. American Journal of Industrial Medicine 48:491–502.

Eaton, A. and Nocerino, T. (2000) The effectiveness of Health and Committees: Results of a survey of public sector workplaces. Industrial Relations 39:265–290.

Eijkemans, G. J. and Takala, J. (2005) Moving knowledge of global burden into preventive action. American Journal of Industrial Medicine 48:395–399.

Forst, L., Nickels, L. and Conroy, L. (2009) The WHO modules in occupational safety and health: training for prevention. Public Health Reports 124(1):169–176.

Garcie-Herrero, S. (2012) Working conditions, Psychological, physical symptoms and occupational accidents. Bayesian Network Models, Safety Science 50(9):1760–1774.

Gunningham, N. (1999) Integrating management systems and occupational health and safety regulation. Journal of Law and Society 26(2):192–214.

Gunningham, N. (2005) Safety, regulation and the mines inspectorate: Lessons from Western Australia. Journal of Occupational Health and Safety 21(4):299.

Hernberg, S. (1992) Introduction to Occupational Epidemiology. Philadelphia: Lewis Publishers.

IAEA, ILO, WHO. (1998) Health Surveillance of Persons Occupationally Exposed to Ionizing Radiation: Guidance for Occupational Physicians, Safety Reports Series No. 5. Vienna: IAEA, ILO, WHO.

IAEA. (1999) Assessment of Occupational Exposure due to External Sources of Radiation IAEA Safety Standards, Series No. RS-G-1.3. Vienna: International Atomic Energy Agency.

IAEA. (1999) Occupational Radiation Protection IAEA Safety Standards, Series No. RS-G-1.1. Vienna: International Atomic Energy Agency.

ILO. (1993) Your Health and Safety at work: Chemicals in the Workplace. Geneva: International Labour Organization.

ILO. (1996) Your Health and Safety at Work: Instructor's Guide to the Modules. Geneva: International Labour Organization.

ILO. (1996) Your Health and Safety at Work: Male and Female Reproductive Health Hazards in the Workplace. Geneva: International Labour Organization.

ILO. (1996) Your Health and Safety at Work: Controlling Hazards. Geneva: International Labour Organization.

ILO. (1996) Your Health and Safety at Work: Health and Safety for Women and Children. Geneva: International Labour Organization.

ILO. (1996) Your Health and Safety at Work: Using Health and Safety Committees at Work. Geneva: International Labour Organization.

ILO. (1998) Safety and Health in the Use of Chemicals at Work: A Training Manual. Geneva: International Labour Organization.

ILO. (2001) Ambient Factors in the Workplace: An ILO Code of Practice. Geneva: International Labour Organization.

Jonathan, G. K. and Rosemary, W. M. (2016) Maintaining health and safety at workplace: Employee and employer's role in ensuring a safe working environment. International University Journal of Education and Practice 7(29):1–7.

Leigh, J., Macaskill, P., Kuosma, E. and Mandryk, J. (1999) Global burden of disease and injury due to occupational factors. Epidemiology 10:626–631.

Levy, B. S. and Wegman, D. H. (1994) Occupational Health: Recognizing and Preventing Work-Related Disease. Boston: Little Brown.

Liu, K. (2019) Regulating health and safety at the workplace: Prescriptive approach vs goal-oriented approach. Safety Science 120:950–961.
Magalhães, L. M. C. A., *et al.* (2022) A study on occupational health and safety. BMC Public Health 22:2186.
Muthuviknesh, R. and Kumar, K. A. (2014) The effect of occupational health and safety management on work environment: A prospective study. International Journal of Advance Research in Computer Science and Management Studies 2(6):904–909.
Palali, A. and Van Ours, J. C. (2017) Workplace accidents and workplace safety: On under-reporting and temporary jobs. Labour 31(1):1–14.
Qasim, M., Bashir, A., Shan, A. and Anees, M. M. (2014) Concept of occupational health and safety and evaluation of awareness level among employees. World Applied Sciences Journal 32(5):904–909.
Rajgopal, T. (2000) Occupational health in India—current and future perspective. Journal of Indian Medical Association 98:432–433.
Reilly, B., Paci, P. and Holl, P. (1995) Unions, safety committees and workplace injuries. British Journal of Industrial Relations 33(2):273–288.
Rosenstock, L. and Cullen, M. R. (1994) Textbook of Clinical Occupational and Environmental Medicine. Philadelphia: Saunders.
Sánchez, F. A. S., Peláez, G. I. C. and Alí, J. C. S. (2017) Occupational safety and health in construction: A review of applications and trends. Industrial Health 55:210–218.
Schulman, P. R. (2020) Organizational structure and safety culture: Conceptual and practical challenges. Safety Science 126.
Stout, N. A. and Linn, H. I. (2002) Occupational injury prevention research: Progress and priorities. Injury Prevention 8:9–14.
Suparna, N. S. and Jaiswal, A. (2021) The occupational health and safety. Anthropo-Indialogs 1(3):261–269.
WHO. (2005) Occupational Health. Geneva, Switzerland: World Health Organization.
WHO. (2011) Global Status Report on Non-communicable Diseases 2010. Geneva: World Health Organization.

8 Waterborne Diseases

"The Truly Healthy environment is not merely safe but stimulating"

—William H. Stewart

FACT FILE

According to the World Health Organization:

- More than two billion people live in water-stressed nations, which are likely to get worsen due to increasing population and climate change
- Nearly two billion people around the globe are using the contaminated drinking water, faecal matter being the most important microbial contaminant resulting in poor health outcome
- Arsenic, fluoride/nitrate, together with pollutants like hydraulic fracturing chemicals, pharmaceuticals, pesticides, and micro-plastics not only acts as the chemical hazards to drinking water but pose threats to public health
- Safe and adequate water enables practicing hygiene, which is a key measure to prevent diarrhoeal diseases, acute respiratory infections and many other ignored tropical diseases
- Microbial contamination of drinking water is responsible for transmission of various diseases, viz. diarrhoea, dysentery, cholera, typhoid, and polio with estimated more than 485,000 diarrhoeal deaths each year**
- In 2020, 5.8 billion people across the global used a securely handled drinking-water service – viz. one located on premises, available when essential, and free from pollution
- About 2 billion people are deprived of safely managed services including 1.2 billion people with a better water source situated within a round trip of 30 minutes
- About 282 million people are living with inadequate services, or a better-quality water source demanding more than 30 minutes to fetch water
- 368 million people across the globe consume water from unprotected wells and springs
- 122 million people gather untreated surface water from natural lakes, ponds, rivers and streams
- More than 829,000 people die each year because of diarrhoea caused by unsafe drinking-water, sanitation, and poor hygiene
- Nearly 297,000 children under 5 years die due to diarrhoea which is preventable by addressing the risk factors

DOI: 10.1201/9781003464785-8

- Waterborne diseases are believed to be of public health concern and have the potential of causing large outbreaks
- Waterborne diseases are responsible for causing high disease burden owing to the large number of cases and deaths, particularly in young children
- For many waterborne diseases no specific treatment is available, for instance, hepatitis E.
- The anti-microbial drug resistance is increasing for some bacterial diseases
- By 2020, 54 percent of the global population used a safely managed sanitation service
- Over 1.7 billion people still don't have basic sanitation services, viz. private toilets or latrines
- 494 million still defecate in the open, viz. in street gutters, behind bushes or open water bodies
- In 2020, 45 percent of the household wastewater generated globally was discharged without safe treatment
- Nearly 10 percent of the world's population is believed to consume food irrigated by wastewater
- Poor sanitation decreases the human health and hampers the socio-economic development

As per the reports of World Health Organization by 2015:

- 71 percent of the global population used a safely managed drinking water service, specifically, one located in the premises, readily available and free from contamination
- Assessment for safely managed drinking water was available for 96 countries, i.e. 35 percent of the global population
- One out of three people using safely managed drinking water services lived in rural areas
- Eight out of ten people used better-quality water sources
- Three out of four people used improved sources located free from contamination
- 844 million people still lacked even a basic drinking water service
- 263 million people spent over 30 minutes per round trip to collect water from an improved source
- 159 million people still collect drinking water directly from surface water sources
- 39 percent of the global population (2.9 billion people) used a safely managed sanitation service
- Estimates for safely managed sanitation were available for 84 countries, i.e. 48 percent of the global population
- Two out of five people using safely managed sanitation services lived in rural areas
- 27 percent of the global population used private sanitation facilities linked to drains from which wastewater was treated

- 13 percent of global population used toilets or latrines where excreta were disposed of *in situ*
- 68 percent of the global population used at least a basic sanitation service
- 2.3 billion people still lack even a basic sanitation service and 600 million people used a limited sanitation service, i.e. improved facilities shared with other households
- 892 million people worldwide still practice open defecation
- 70 countries had comparable data available on hand washing with soap and water, representing 30 percent of the global population
- In least developed countries, 27 percent of the population had basic hand washing facilities with soap and water, whereas 26 percent had hand washing facilities lacking soap or water. The remaining 47 percent had no facility
- High-income countries lack sufficient data to estimate the population with basic hand washing facilities
- Incidence of disease can be stopped by providing safe water supply, adequate sanitation services and better hygiene practices
- Diarrhoeal disease alone accounts to an estimated 3.6 percent of the total DALY global burden of disease and is responsible for the deaths of 1.5 million people every year
- It is estimated that 58 percent or 842,000 deaths per year is attributable to unsafe water supply, sanitation and hygiene and includes 361,000 deaths of children under age five, mostly in low-income countries
- Adequate water, sanitation and hygiene play an important role in preventing many more diseases, improving nutritional outcomes and provision of quality care in healthcare settings
- More than 50 percent urban people in developing countries are still affected at one time or another by diseases related to insufficient access to safe drinking-water and improved sanitation
- Internationally, 26 percent of people drink water contaminated with faecal indicator bacteria
- Contaminated water can transmit diseases such as diarrhoea, cholera, dysentery, typhoid and polio
- Health risks are worsened by poor sanitation
- Urban solid waste disposal is another sanitation-related challenge
- Recent estimates suggest that cities generate 1.3 billion tonnes of solid waste per year, a figure expected to rise to 2.2 billion tonnes by 2025.

8.1 INTRODUCTION

Access to safe drinking water and hygienic living environment are not only the basic rights of all living organisms but the prerequisites for realizing the goals of sustainable development, including health, food security, and poverty reduction. Water-related ecosystems are indispensable to life and have always offered natural premises for flourishing of human civilizations, with advantages, for instance, conveyance, natural cleansing, irrigation, flood fortification and place for biodiversity to flourish. Water quality is one of the important global concerns for the reason that drinking water sources are under the increasing threats of contamination, with far-reaching health penalties, which the children are paying. Not only this, the polluted water sources are spreading the diseases caused through skin contact or by vectors. Besides direct health implications, the unfit drinking water has a number of subtle or indirect adverse health effects. The children enfeebled by recurrent incidents of diarrhoea are more prone to be seriously affected by malnutrition, leaving them physically stunted for entire life. Chronic consumption of unsafe drinking water is believed to cause permanent cognitive damage and moreover the people with compromised immune systems, for instance, those with HIV and AIDS are unable to resist or recover from the waterborne diseases. The magnitude of poor water quality goes beyond health. Chronic spells of waterborne diseases impose significant socio-economic burdens both on the fatalities and the society as a whole.

The increasing population, intensification of farming and allied activities, expansion of urban and industrial areas is overpowering and undermining nature's ability to realize the key roles and deliver basic services. The challenges of meeting the growing needs of water in a justifiable way are formidable, but these can be incapacitated. The execution of integrated water resources management, including the trans-boundary level and mainstreaming water and sanitation in the policies and programmes is imperative. The topographical, sociocultural and economic disparities exist, not only between rural and urban areas but in towns and cities where the people belonging to low-income, informal or unlawful suburb hamlets usually have limited access to quality drinking-water as compared to the other inhabitants.

8.2 WATER: THE ELIXIR OF LIFE

Water (of other areas) is the basis of entire life on planet earth. All living organisms have a huge amount of water in their body, and water plays a significant role in all life processes. Likewise, the moisture in the soil is vital for the growth of plants. The main sources of water are rain and snowfall. Much of farming depends on seasonal rainfall and is affected by its failure or irregularity. Chemically, water is composed of hydrogen and oxygen elements and exists in gaseous, liquid, and solid states. Clouds are composed of suspended droplets of water and ice. Steam or water vapour is the gaseous state of water. It is the most abundant substance on earth and about 71 percent of the earth's surface is covered with water in form of oceans and seas (about 96.5 percent) as groundwater (1.7 percent), in glaciers and the ice caps (1.7 percent), and in air as vapour, clouds (0.001 percent). Water constantly moves through hydrological cycle as evaporation, condensation, precipitation, and runoff. Being polar inorganic compound, water is tasteless and odourless liquid at room temperature and known as *universal solvent* or *solvent of life* for its ability to dissolve many substances. Water molecules form hydrogen bonds with each other and are strongly polar. The polarity of water permits it to disassociate ions in salts and attach to other polar substances, for instance, alcohols and acids, thus dissolving them. It has relatively high boiling point of 100 °C. Water is amphoteric, and can exhibit properties of an acid or a base, depending on the pH of the solution.

Due to its amphoteric nature, it undergoes self-ionization. Diseases owing to poor access to drinking-water, unimproved sanitation, and poor hygiene practices result in four percent deaths and 5.7 percent disabilities or ill health. About 80 percent of urban inhabitants have access to piped drinking water and 96 percent have access to improved drinking water sources. But, the microbiological condition of water remains poor.

Social inequalities play an important role in water and sanitation-related risks – with informal settlements and slums usually having lower levels of access than other parts of the city. Slums and other densely populated areas pose threats for improving the sanitation. Extension of urban areas also makes setting up of sewage infrastructure more expensive as compared to planned, compact development. Water safety and quality are essential to human development and health. Providing access to safe water is one of the most effective means of encouraging health and reducing poverty.

Being an international authority on public health and water quality, WHO efforts to prevent transmission of waterborne disease remained significant. This is realized by encouraging health-based rules to governments and working in partnership to encourage effective risk management practices to water suppliers, public, and residential areas. Safe water, sanitation, and hygiene (together known as WASH) are vital for human health and safety. However, millions of people worldwide lacks adequate safe water, sanitation and hygiene services and therefore suffer from or are exposed to a variety of avoidable diseases. Lack of safe water, sanitation and hygiene adversely affects quality of life and weakens the fundamental human rights. Poor safe water, sanitation and hygiene services also deteriorate health systems, pose threats to health security and place a heavy pressure on economies.

Drinking water, even from an established and properly managed source, is not really free of faecal pathogens and safe for health. Drinking water sources undergo contamination and require suitable treatment to eliminate disease-causing impurities. Contamination of drinking water can occur at source water or distribution system after water treatment. The sources of water contamination include naturally occurring chemicals and minerals, fertilizers, pesticides, and sewer overflows or wastewater releases. The toxins in water can cause adverse health effects, including gastro-intestinal illness, reproductive problems, and neurological disorders. Infants, young children, pregnant women, elderly, and people with weak immune system are particularly vulnerable to illness.

8.2.1 Defining Water Quality

The physical, chemical, and biological characteristics of water define its quality and based on its source, water can be classified as groundwater and surface water. Both types of water are exposed to risk of pollution from farming, industrial, and domestic activities; the key pollutants being the heavy metals, pesticides, fertilizers, hazardous chemicals, and oils. It can also be classified as-potable water, palatable water, polluted water, and infected water. While the potable water is safe to drink, has pleasant taste, and can be used for domestic purpose;

TABLE 8.1
Water Quality Parameters

Physical Parameters	Chemical Parameters	Biological Parameters
Turbidity, colour, taste and odour, solids, temperature, electrical conductivity (EC)	pH, acidity, alkalinity, chloride, sulphate, nitrogen, fluoride, iron and manganese, copper and zinc, hardness, dissolved oxygen (DO), biochemical oxygen demand (BOD), Chemical oxygen demand (COD), toxic inorganic/organic substances and radioactive substances	Bacteria, Algae, Viruses, and Protozoa

the palatable water is aesthetically pleasing but contain chemicals which are not harmful to living organism. But the contaminated or polluted water contain undesirable physical, chemical, biological, or radiological substances, which make water unfit for drinking or domestic use. The infected water is polluted with pathogens, which can cause diseases. There are three quality parameters of water physical, chemical, and biological, which are discussed in detail in the subsequent section (Table 8.1).

8.2.2 Physico-chemical Properties of Water

A. **Physical Properties**

Turbidity: It is the cloudiness of water and is a measure of the ability of light to pass through water. It is caused by suspended material such as clay, silt, organic material, plankton, and other particulate materials in water. Turbidity in drinking water is usually unacceptable. Turbidity increases the cost of water treatment, while the particulate matter provides hiding space for harmful microorganisms. The suspended materials can clog or damage fish gills, reducing its confrontation to diseases, decreasing its growth rates, affecting egg, and larval maturing. These particles also provide adsorption media for heavy metals, such as, Hg, Cr, Pb, etc. and many hazardous organic pollutants and pesticides. High turbidity increases the temperature of water because the suspended particles absorb more sun heat and decreases the concentration of dissolved oxygen.

Temperature: It affects the taste, thickness, solubility, odours, and chemical reactions. The sedimentation, chlorination, and Biological Oxygen Demand (BOD) are dependent on temperature and it also affects the biosorption process of dissolved heavy metals in water.

Colour: The materials from organic matter, viz. vegetation and inorganic matter, for instance, soil, stones, and rocks impart colour to water, which is unpleasant for aesthetic reasons.

Taste and Odour: Taste and odour in water is resultant of foreign matter, such as, organic materials, inorganic compounds, or dissolved gasses which originate from natural, domestic, or agricultural processes.

Solids: Solids in water occur either in solution or in suspension, which can be identified by using a glass fibre filter that the water sample passes through. The suspended solids are retained at the top of the filter and the dissolved solids pass through the filter along with water.

Total Solids: It is a measure of the suspended and dissolved solids in water. Suspended solids are those that can be held on a water filter and are capable of settling out the water column onto the stream bottom when stream velocities are low.

Total Dissolved Solids (TDS): It is the amount of organic and inorganic materials, such as metals, minerals, salts, and ions, dissolved in a particular volume of water. TDS are basically a quantity of anything dissolved in water that is not an H_2O molecule.

Total Suspended Solids: It is the amount of fine particulate matter that remains in suspension in water. It provides an actual weight of particulate matter in a given volume of sample.

Electrical Conductivity (EC): It is a measure of the capacity of a solution to carry or conduct an electrical current. Since the electrical current is carried by ions in solution, the conductivity increases when the concentration of ions increases. Therefore, it is one of the main factors which determines the suitability of water for irrigation and fire fighting.

Specific Heat: Water has high specific heat, i.e. 4.18 J/g C^o.

High Heat Capacity: Lots of energy is required to raise the temperature of water by a degree, so it helps in regulating the temperature in the environment.

Polarity: Water molecules are polar with partial positive charge on the hydrogen, and a partial negative charge on the oxygen with a bent overall structure.

High heat of vaporization: Water gets converted from its liquid form to gaseous state when the heat of vaporization is attained. Sweat contains water and the evaporating water absorbs excess body heat and has cooling effect.

Cohesive and adhesive properties: Water molecules have strong cohesive forces owing to their capacity to form hydrogen bonds with one another. These forces are accountable for surface tension. Water has adhesive properties which allow it to adhere to other substances.

B. Chemical Properties

pH: pH, one of the most important parameters of water quality, is defined as the negative logarithm of the hydrogen ion concentration. Being a dimensionless number, it indicates the strength of an acidic or a basic solution. It measures the acidity or basicity of water. Acidic water contains extra hydrogen ions (H^+) and basic water contains extra hydroxyl (OH^-) ions. pH ranges from 0 to 14, 7 being the neutral. pH less than 7 indicates acidic nature, while pH greater than 7 indicates a basic solution. Pure water is neutral, with a pH close to 7.0 at 25°C. Owing to atmospheric CO_2 gas, normal rainfall has a pH of nearly 5.6. Safe range of pH for drinking water is from 6.5 to 8.5. A high pH imparts bitter taste and decreases the efficacy of chlorine disinfection. The amount of oxygen in water increases as pH rises. Low-pH of water is responsible for corrosion of metals and other substances. Pollution modifies the pH of water, which is harmful for aquatic plants and animals.

Even the moderately acidic water affects the hatching of fish eggs, affect the fish gills and damage membranes. Extremely high or low pH can kill most fishes. Likewise, amphibians are extremely endangered by low pH for their skin is sensitive to pollutants. Heavy metals dissolve more easily in highly acidic water because the heavy metals become much more toxic when dissolved in water. A change in the pH affects the presence of chemicals in water.

Acidity: Acidity is the measure of acids in a solution. It is the quantitative capacity to neutralize a strong base to a selected pH level. Acidity in water is due to CO_2, mineral acids, and hydrolysed salts. Acids affect diverse processes like corrosion, chemical reactions and biological activities. Atmospheric CO_2 or CO_2 due to respiration of aquatic organisms makes the water acidic due to the formation of carbonic acid (H_2CO_3).

Alkalinity: The alkalinity of water is defined as its capacity to neutralize its acidity. Alkalinity of water is due to the presence of hydroxide ions (OH^-), bicarbonate ions (HCO_3^-), and carbonate ions (CO_3^{2-}), or a mixture of two of these ions in water. The high level of acidity or alkalinity in water is indicative of industrial or chemical pollution. The natural phenomenon occurring in water, for instance, volcanoes causes alkalinity or acidity. The acidity and alkalinity in natural water offers a buffering action that protects fish and other aquatic organisms from sudden changes in pH.

Chloride: Chloride occurs naturally in groundwater, streams, and lakes, but the presence of moderately high concentration of chloride in freshwater is indicative of pollution. Rocks containing chloride, farm runoff, and wastewater are the main sources of chlorides. Presence of chloride ions in drinking water has no adverse impact on public health, but higher concentration impart an unpleasant salted taste. Optimum level of chloride is essential for normal functioning of cell both in animals and plants. The standard chloride level for public drinking water should not exceed 250 mg/L.

Sulphate: Sulphate ions (SO_4^{2-}) occur both in natural and wastewater. The high concentration of sulphate in natural water is due to leaching of natural deposits of sodium or magnesium sulphate. High concentration of sulphate ions in drinking water not only affects its taste but may have laxative effects.

Nitrogen: Nitrogen occurs in four different forms in both normal and wastewater. These are organic nitrogen, ammonia nitrogen, nitrite nitrogen, and nitrate nitrogen. If water is polluted due to sewage, most of the nitrogen is in the form of organic and ammonia, which is changed to nitrites and nitrates by the microbial action. Nitrogen in the form of nitrate acts as a basic nutrient which is responsible for the growth of plants. Higher concentration of nitrate in surface water accelerates the rapid growth of algae which worsens the water quality. Nitrates released from chemical fertilizers mixes with the groundwater. Excessive nitrate concentration in drinking water has immediate and severe health impacts on infants. The nitrate ions react with blood haemoglobin, and reduce blood's ability to retain oxygen which can cause the diseases, viz. blue baby or methemoglobinemia.

Fluoride: An adequate amount of fluoride ions (F^-) in drinking water is good for dental health. About 1.0 mg/L is effective in preventing tooth decay, mainly among children but excessive amount of fluoride causes discolouring of, a condition defined as dental fluorosis. The permissible level of fluoride in public water supplies is governed by the local climate. In the warmer areas, the maximum permissible level of fluoride for potable water is 1.4 mg/L, while in cold climates it is up to 2.4 mg/L.

Iron and Manganese: Though presence of iron (Fe) and manganese (Mn) in water don't have any health implications, yet these impart a bitter taste to water even at very low concentration. Both the metals occur in groundwater in form of ferrous (Fe^{2+}) and manganous (Mn^{2+}) ions. Once these come in contact with air, they form the insoluble ferric (Fe^{3+}) and manganic (Mn^{3+}) forms which make the water muddy and undesirable.

Copper and Zinc: In small concentrations, copper (Cu) and zinc (Zn) are non-toxic but these are vital and useful not only for human health but for the growth of plants and animals. In high concentration, these impart an undesirable taste to drinking water.

Hardness: The term hardness conveys the properties of extremely mineralized waters. The dissolved minerals in water results in deposition of the same in hot water pipes, and hampers the making of lather with soap. Calcium and magnesium ions released from the rocks and soil is responsible for the hardness in natural water. These ions are present as bicarbonates, sulphates, and at times as chlorides and nitrates.

Normally, surface water is less hard than the groundwater. The hardness is of two types – temporary hardness, due to carbonates and bicarbonates, which can be removed by boiling, and permanent hardness caused by sulphates and chlorides and persists even after boiling. Water with more than 300 mg/L of hardness is believed to be hard, and hardness more than 150 mg/L is perceptible. The water having hardness less than 75 mg/L is regarded as soft. From health point of view, hardness up to 500 mg/L is harmless, but higher than the permissible limit has a laxative effect.

Dissolved Oxygen: It is one of the most important water quality parameters especially in context of natural water sources. It is an important test of water pollution; the more is the concentration of dissolved oxygen, the better will be the quality of water. To some extent, O_2 is soluble in water and is quite sensitive to temperature. The amount of dissolved O_2 varies depending on pressure, temperature, and salinity. Dissolved O_2 doesn't have direct health implications, but drinking water with very little or no O_2 tastes unpleasant.

Biochemical Oxygen Demand (BOD): Bacteria and other microorganisms utilize organic substances for preparing food. O_2 is consumed when the microbes metabolize organic material to simpler compounds, such as CO_2 and H_2O, and the energy so released is utilized by the microbes for growth and reproduction. If this process takes place in water, the oxygen used up is the Dissolved Oxygen (DO) in the water. When O_2 is not substituted constantly by natural or artificial means, the concentration of DO will reduce and the microbes start decomposing the organic materials. This call for oxygen is known as Biochemical Oxygen Demand (BOD). The more is the organic material in water; the microbes will use higher BOD. The microbes take about 20 days to completely decompose the organic material. The quantity of O_2 used in a specified volume of water to completely decay or stabilize all biodegradable organic substances is called the ultimate BOD or BODL.

Chemical Oxygen Demand (COD): This parameter measures all organics, viz. the biodegradable and the non-biodegradable substances.

Toxic Inorganic Substances: Though in traces, numerous inorganic toxic substances are found in water and can threaten the public health. Some of these are drawn from the natural sources but others are released due to industrial activities and/or improper management of hazardous waste. Toxic inorganic substances may be metallic compounds, viz. Cd, Cr, Pb, Hg, Ag, As, Ba, etc., which can result in acute fatal poisoning or may cause chronic diseases; these may be non-metallic compounds, including nitrates (NO^{3-}) and cyanides (CN^-). Cyanide causes oxygen deficiency by attaching itself with the haemoglobin thereby hampering the O_2 carrying capacity of RBCs, thus causing cyanosis or blue skin syndrome. It also affects CNS and functioning of thyroid gland.

Toxic Organic Substances: More than 100 toxic organic compounds are found in water. They are not found naturally in water, but are released due to anthropogenic activities. The insecticides, pesticides, solvents, detergents, and disinfectants are the main sources of toxic organic compounds.

Radioactive Material: Radioactive substances are released in water in form of wastes from the nuclear power plants, industries, or medical research institutes using radioactive chemicals and mining of radioactive materials. During their decay, they release beta, alpha, and gamma radiation and exposure to these radioactive substances causes genetic and somatic diseases.

C. **Biological Parameters**

One of the most important indicators of water quality is the presence or absence of living organisms. Species Diversity Index (SDI) through fish and insect life helps in assessing the water quality. Many organisms can act as indicators for presence of pollutants. Microbes are present everywhere in nature and human body has a normal population of microbes in the intestinal tract, a big portion of which is made of coliform bacteria. Although there are millions of microbes per millilitre in wastewater, but most of these are harmless. Water becomes harmful only when the wastewater contains wastes released by the people infected with diseases.

Bacteria: Under favourable conditions, bacteria can reproduce rapidly. Their categorization is done on the basis of metabolism of food. Bacteria that require oxygen for metabolism are called aerobic bacteria, while those living in an oxygen-free environment are called anaerobic bacteria. There are some facultative bacteria, which can live either in the absence or presence of oxygen.

At low temperature, bacteria grow and reproduce gradually. As the temperature increases, the rate of growth and reproduction doubles. The majority of bacteria live in an optimal temperature of about 35°C. A number of serious waterborne diseases are caused by bacteria, namely, typhoid and paratyphoid fever, shigellosis, and cholera.

Algae: Algae are mainly nuisance organisms for the taste and odour problems they create. Some species of algae cause serious environmental and public health problems, for example, blue-green algae can kill cattle and other domestic animals if they happen to drink water containing blue-green algae.

Viruses: Viruses are parasites that need a host to live and can pass through filters that do not permit the passage of bacteria. Waterborne viral pathogens are known to cause infectious hepatitis and poliomyelitis. Most of the waterborne viruses can be deactivated by the disinfection process conducted in the water treatment plant.

Protozoa: Protozoa, the single-celled microscopic animal are free-floating in water are called zooplanktons. They form cysts that are difficult to inactivate by disinfection. They are responsible for causing numerous waterborne protozoan diseases.

Indicator organisms: Coliforms are important biological indicators of water and pollution. They are present in the intestinal tract of humans, and millions are excreted with body wastes. Water contaminated with sewage contains coliforms. *E. coli* is the most common form of bacteria and about 3 million *E. coli* is found in 100 ml untreated sewage. Coliforms are hostile organisms and survive in the water longer than most other pathogens and can cause numerous diseases.

8.3 WATER AND HUMAN HEALTH

Water is the basic compound required for the functioning of all life forms that exist on earth. Water is the reason behind earth and is the only planet that supports life. Water is a universal solvent, and it is difficult to imagine the functioning of life processes without water. In body, water acts as a lubricant during the digestion of food. Water in saliva helps in chewing and swallowing food. Food goes down into the alimentary tract with the help of water. The functions of body's cells and organs depend on water. Water is involved in carrying valuable nutrients around the body in the blood. In digestive tract, the nutrients break down and carried to the site where these are required in the body. Water helps in getting rid of harmful toxins and wastes through urination and perspiration and thus reducing constipation. Drinking sufficient water supports body organs to get rid of toxins. Water regulates body temperature through perspiration by producing a cooling effect. Water for human use must be pleasant and safe to drink, i.e. totally clear and free from taste, smell and colour. Safe drinking water or the potable water does not contain unsafe or potentially harmful substances and doesn't pose any threat to human health. The unsafe substances could be microbes or chemicals. Unsafe water results in bad health for people of all age groups. However, some people including infants and young children, older people are at greater risk. Water constitutes about 70 percent of human weight and blood alone contains approximately 82 percent water and human brain is made up of about 95 percent water. Losing only 2 percent of water can cause dehydration. Water plays an important role in keeping environment clean. It is vital for personal hygiene and is used to wash hands and bodies, wash places, such as, toilets that could probably have harmful microbes. Food is prepared with water and many foods naturally contain large amounts of water, e.g. milk contains nearly 88 percent water; eggs contain 66 percent, fish 80 percent, and potatoes 75 percent of water.

8.3.1 Importance of Water in Body

Water is next to oxygen with regard to its significance in the body. Water constitutes about 67 to 75 percent of the total body weight. Water is involved in all body processes. It is an efficient heat conductor and helps to maintain the uniform body temperature. It acts as a protector of internal organs. Water is essential and acts as a cushion which prevents the transmission of shock. Water acts as a solvent for various chemical compounds and as a medium for occurrence of bio-chemical reactions. Inside cells, water is a part of the intracellular fluid besides its presence outside cells. It is a part of the extracellular fluid, which is further divided into interstitial fluid, present between cells and inter-vascular fluid, i.e. water in the bloodstream. Water moves liberally from one compartment to another and constitutes a majority of body's weight involving in various life processes, including:

- Removal of waste from the body
- Regulation of body temperature
- Helping in the functioning of the brain

TABLE 8.2
Importance of Water in Body

Absorption of nutrients	Water helps in dissolving vitamins, minerals, and other nutrients from food and their absorption
Boosting Energy	Water activates body's metabolism, which has positive impact on energy level
Circulation of oxygen in blood	Water carries useful nutrients and oxygen to entire body
Digestion	Water helps in digestion of food, for it is required not only for the bowel movement, but functioning of various enzymes, electrolytes and hormones
Excretion	H_2O helps to excrete waste through perspiration, urination, and defecation in form of sweat, urine, and faecal matter
Fighting illnesses	Drinking water helps in managing constipation, renal stones, exercise-induced asthma, urinary tract infection, hypertension
Formation of saliva	Water is the main constituent of saliva, which helps in breaking down solid food and functioning of electrolytes, mucus, and enzymes
Healthy skin	Sufficient water intake keeps the skin hydrated and promote the formation of collagen
Improving cognitive function and mood	Water prevents dehydration, which may result in fatigue, confusion and anxiety
Maximize physical performance	Water is essential during physical activity, for hydration affects the strength, power, and endurance
Prevents constipation	Water together with magnesium and fibre helps in regulating the bowel movements
Prevents dehydration	Water prevents dehydration thereby preventing swelling of brain, kidney failure, and seizures
Lubricant	Water lubricates and cushions the joints, spinal cord, and tissues help in the physical activity thereby lessening the problem caused by immobility of joints
Regulate body temperature	Water helps in regulating the body temperature and electrolyte balance. Sweat regulates the body temperature

Water is involved in various life processes, some of the important function of water are listed in the Table 8.2.

8.4 SANITATION AND HEALTH-RELATED CHALLENGES

Environmental sanitation envisions elevation of health of the community by offering clean environment and ending or interrupting the cycle of disease. It depends on various factors including:

- Availability of resources
- Capacity building in related areas

- Cultural factors related to sanitation
- Hygiene of people
- Judicial processes
- Political obligation
- Progressive and appropriate know-hows in accordance to community's need
- Social factors including community's behavioural pattern
- Socioeconomic development of a country

India still lags behind in the field of environmental sanitation. The unhygienic environments are terrible in India and require a great sanitary awakening. Improvement in sanitation needs innovative policies and direct interventions with follow-up assessment. The need of the hour is to recognize the present system of sanitation with regard to its structure and working and to place in order the need-based control policies. These priorities are mainly significant owing to the issue of water limitations, environment-related health issues, rapid population growth, unequal distribution of water resources, administrative problems, urbanization and industrialization, migration of people, and fast economic growth. Sectoral demands for water are increasing fast in India mainly due to urbanization and it is assessed that by 2025, more than 50 percent of people will live in cities and towns. Population increase, growing incomes, and industrial development are accountable for this dramatic change. National Urban Sanitation Policy of 2008 was framed to quickly encourage sanitation in urban areas. As part of its National Urban Sanitation Policy, Ministry of Urban Development commissioned the survey in November 2008. The sanitation and health challenges are:

1. Stopping of water pollution
2. Increasing water shortage and prospective for water recycle and management
3. Executing ground-breaking low-cost sanitation system
4. Offering viable water supplies and sanitation in urban and semi-urban areas
5. Decreasing inequalities within the states
6. Sustainability of water and sanitation services

Thus, state-of-the-art methods are vital to safeguard the accessibility of low-cost, simple, and locally suitable water, sanitation interventions and incorporating these methods in prevailing social institutions, for instance, schools, markets, and healthcare amenities. Sanitation is one of the prerequisite of a healthy, contented and respectable life. However, the reality for billions of people is the polluted environments. Sanitation is a human right. Everybody is entitled to avail sanitation services that offer privacy, confirm self-respect and security, and that are considerably available and rational. Sanitation is a public good, offering societal benefits, improved health and contributes to socio-economic development. The absence of safe sanitation causes illness and disease that affect the vulnerable section of society. Poor sanitation affects entire community, especially the vulnerable and underprivileged, mainly women and people with disabilities. Sanitation workers, often defamed and downgraded, face offensive health risks and shame in an unregulated environment. Investment in governance, funding, capacity building, data and information, and innovation can act as a pathway for realizing the universal and safe sanitation for all. Sanitation is vital to health, child development, and socioeconomic progress. The lack of safe sanitation leads to a variety of adverse health impacts, including:

- Diarrhoea, the main health concern and an important cause of disease and death among children under five years of age in low and middle-income countries.
- Cholera, an acute diarrhoeal disease that can be fatal if left unattended.
- Neglected tropical diseases, for example, soil-transmitted helminthic infections, which at global level account for a substantial burden of disease.
- Vector-borne diseases such as West Nile virus or lymphatic filariasis
- Stunting affecting nearly one-quarter of children under five years of age worldwide and manifests in form of recurrent diarrhoea, helminthic infections, and environmental enteric dysfunction related to unhygienic settings, leading to low physical and cognitive development
- Antimicrobial resistance, by increasing the risk of avoidable infections that can be treated with antibiotics and by dispersal of resistant organisms in the environment though unmanaged wastewater and sludge.

Insufficient sanitation contributes directly or indirectly – by polluting drinking-water and hands to nearly 830,000 deaths, over 49 million DALYs due to diarrhoeal diseases and many more from other diseases and conditions including soil-transmitted helminth infections, malnutrition, trachoma, lymphatic filariasis, etc. and diseases linked with poor wastewater management practices. In addition to the economic costs, lack of sanitation has negative impacts that cannot be easily quantified. Impacts on dignity, poverty, infirmity, safety, gender, and education denote unrealized human potential and are borne by the most vulnerable and disadvantaged. The ability to manage the functioning of body, including urination, defecation, and menstruation, is at the core of dignity. Lack of public utilities compels people to resort to open defecation, and in turn is the greatest threat to dignity. Similarly, poorly-managed shared sanitation facilities increase the risk of exposure to numerous diseases and infections.

The health of poor is extremely affected by lack of sanitation. Proper sanitary facilities are lacking in rural areas. Poor and marginalized groups live '*downstream*', making them prone to the effects of unmanaged faecal waste. People with disabilities suffer insults to their dignity due to lack of appropriate sanitation services. Poor access to sanitation services threatens the security and exposes vulnerable groups – mainly women and girls – to sexual, psychosomatic, and physical violence. Poor sanitation increases health risks specifically among women; for instance, women suffering from worm infestation and other diseases become anaemic and undernourished, increasing the risk of maternal death. Lack of adequate sanitation facilities at workplace discourages women from seeking employment. Likewise, lack of public toilets decreases women's movement and participation in public life and economy. Poor sanitation is known to act as a barrier to school attendance and enrolment in many developing nations, particularly girls after puberty, when their need for management of menstrual hygiene is not addressed.

8.5 WATER-RELATED HEALTH DISORDERS

The majority of water-related health disorders are caused by infectious organisms including pathogenic bacteria, viruses, protozoa, and parasites which attack the body and cause disease. The disease is caused when the infectious agents are swallowed or consumed or else come in contact with human body. The manner in which water comes in contact with human body can be used to categorize the diseases into four main groups.

Safe and easily accessible water is important for public health, whether it is used for drinking, domestic, food production, or recreational purposes. Enhanced water supply and sanitation can boost nations' economic growth and contribute immensely to poverty reduction. In 2010, the UN General Assembly clearly recognized the human right to water and sanitation. Everyone has the right to adequate, constant, safe, tolerable, manageable, and reasonable water for personal and domestic use. Sustainable Development Goals call for universal and impartial access to safe and reasonable drinking water. The target is chased with the indicator of "safely managed drinking water services" – drinking water from a proper water source, free from faecal and chemical contamination. Topographic, sociocultural, and economic disparities persist, not only between rural and urban areas but also in towns and cities where people living in low-income, illegal settlements generally have less access to better-quality sources of drinking-water than other residents. Contaminated water and poor sanitation promote transmission of diseases. Inadequate or inaptly managed water and sanitation services expose people to avoidable health risks. Poor management of urban, industrial, and farm wastewater pollutes the water sources. Presence of naturally occurring minerals, particularly in groundwater, including lead, arsenic, and fluoride, are raised in drinking-water when the leakage from sewerage comes in contact with drinking-water. Insects living or breeding in water carry and transmit various diseases. Some of the insects, known as vectors, prefer breeding in clean, rather than murky water, and household drinking water can offer a better breeding place. The water and sanitation has economic and social implications. Quality water sources mean less expenditure on health, as the people are less likely to fall ill and bear medical costs. Increasing population, water scarcity, climate change, demographic changes and urbanization are posing threats to water supply systems. Over two billion people live in water-stressed nations, which are likely to be worsened as result of climate change and increasing population. Many water-related illnesses rise owing to lack of sufficient clean water for drinking and cooking purposes. Other diseases are caused by poor sanitation and poor personal hygiene practices that are directly linked with the absence of clean water. The two major causes of water-related diseases are:

- **Pollution:** High levels of chemicals, nitrates, and other heavy metals get mixed with water resources because of industrial pollution and/or the overuse of farm chemicals, which badly affects human health.
- **Dirt and Contamination:** Bacteria, viruses, and parasitic organisms contaminate water and cause diseases. Most of the water-related diseases appear after coming in contact with animal or human waste.

Water may carry pathogens of communicable diseases of man or provide the right environment for breeding and propagation of vectors. Moreover, at times the disease causing agent is introduced by human migration. Transmission of disease may be rapid in densely populated areas linked with irrigated lands. Water-related diseases can be alleviated by adopting good engineering practices and appropriate water management. Water-related diseases can be classified into major categories:

1. **Waterborne diseases:** Spread through contaminated drinking water, for instance, diarrhoeal diseases, typhoid fever
2. **Water-washed diseases:** Due to the lack of proper sanitation and hygiene, for instance, Ascariasis (roundworm infection), Ancylostomiasis (hookworm infection)
3. **Water-based diseases:** Transmitted through an aquatic invertebrate organism, for example, Schistosomiasis
4. **Water-related vector-borne diseases:** Transmitted by insects dependent on water for their propagation, for instance, malaria, lymphatic filariasis, onchocerciasis, Japanese encephalitis

8.5.1 Waterborne Diseases

Waterborne diseases are caused by a variety of microbes, bio-toxins, and toxic contaminants, which cause diseases, for instance, cholera, schistosomiasis, and other digestive problems. Outbreaks of waterborne diseases often occur after heavy rainfall/snowfall. Because climate change amplifies the acuteness and incidence of precipitation events, communities-particularly in the developing nations-could be faced with higher disease burden from waterborne diseases. Furthermore, diseases caused by *Vibrio* bacteria, for example, cholera and other gut diseases may pose threat owing to the fact that increasing sea temperature will have impact on the growth and spreading of bacteria. Climate change increases the incidence diarrhoeal disease and life-threatening weather environments may also complicate already-insufficient control efforts. Drought increases the concentrations of effluent pathogens, beating the water treatment plants and polluting surface water. Older water treatment plants are mainly at risk. Changes in ocean and coastal ecosystems, including, the changes in pH, nutrient and pollutant runoff, salinity, and water security degrades fresh water, mainly in areas where people use raw surface water for daily consumption and other activities. Intense extreme weather events cause

TABLE 8.3
List of Waterborne Diseases

Category of Infectious Agent	Disease	Infectious agent
Bacterial	Cholera	*Vibrio cholerae*
	Bacterial dysentery	*Campylobacter jejuni*
	(Acute) gastroenteritis	Various
	Shigellosis	*Shigella* species
	Typhoid fever	*Salmonella typhi*
Viral	Viral gastroenteritis	Rotavirus and others
	Viral hepatitis	Hepatitis A and E viruses
	Poliomyelitis	Polio virus
Protozoal	Amoebic dysentery	*Entamoeba histolytica*
	Cryptosporidiosis	*Cryptosporidium*
	Giardiasis	*Giardia lamblia*
Helminths	Ascariasis (roundworm)	*Ascaris lumbricoides*
	Dracunculiasis (Guinea worm)	*Dracunculus medinensis*
	Trichuriasis (whipworm)	*Trichuris trichiura*

flooding of water and sewage treatment amenities, raising the risk of waterborne diseases.

Ultimately, lack of water causes pressure on farm productivity, crop failure, undernourishment, starvation, population movement, etc. Changes can occur in the distribution and concentration of chemical pollutants in coastal and ocean waters through the release of pollutants earlier locked in polar ice sheets, or in runoff from coastal and watershed development. Waterborne diseases are caused by consumption of water polluted with human or animal faeces containing pathogens. These diseases can be caused by food prepared in water polluted with pathogens. The disease is caused only when the infectious agent enters the body. waterborne diseases include most of the enteric and diarrhoeal diseases caused by bacteria, viruses, protozoa, and helminths (Table 8.3).

Although drinking contaminated water is an important route of transmission for most of the diseases, they may spread by other means, for instance, by consumption of contaminated food. Poor hygiene during food preparation contaminates it. Flies also transmit contamination from faeces to food. If these are swallowed, the probable spreading routes are droplets and aerosols. Touching contaminated surfaces with hands can also be a route for transmission of disease. Some of the common waterborne diseases are:

Arsenicosis: Long-term exposure to low concentration of arsenic in drinking-water causes painful skin keratosis resulting in skin, lungs, bladder, and kidney cancers. Millions of people are possibly in danger due to arsenic poisoning since they rely on water polluted with arsenic and do not have access to safe water or are ignorant about the threats of waterborne diseases.

Causative Agents: Arsenic-contaminated drinking water

Manifestation of Disease: Skin is the main target organ for arsenic toxicity. Skin manifestations of arsenicosis include:

Melanosis: It is hyperpigmentation linked with increased melanin or pigment alteration of the mucosa exhibited by increased melanin pigment in epithelial cells and/or stromal melanophages. Arsenic melanosis is abnormal stimulation of normal melanin biosynthesis by arsenic. Extra-cutaneous manifestations include weakness, anaemia, burning sensation in eyes, inflammation of legs, liver fibrosis, chronic lung disease, gangrene of toes, neuropathy.

Hyperkeratosis: It is a thickening of the outer layer of the skin. The outer layer has a hard, shielding protein called keratin. It causes corns on hands and feet. Arsenical keratosis is a growth of keratin in skin owing to arsenic, which occurs naturally in earth's crust and extensively dispersed in environment. Arsenical compounds are used in industrial, agricultural, and therapeutic purposes. Cutaneous manifestation of arsenicosis is the most distinct change. Non-malignant skin lesions and pigmentary changes are early signs of arsenic toxicity and are main diagnostic standards for arsenicosis. Arsenic may also cause other conditions:

- Bowen's disease
- Cardiovascular diseases
- Developmental abnormalities
- Neurologic and neurobehavioral disorders
- Diabetes
- Hearing impairment
- Hematologic disorders, and
- Various types of cancers

Prophylactic Measures: Ground water is the main source of arsenic poisoning. One of the most effective preventive measures against arsenic poisoning is drinking clean, filtered water and it should be ensured that all foods are cooked in clean water, free from contamination. Those who work in the industries, where the chances of exposure are more, wearing a mask to reduce accidental arsenic inhalation is recommended.

Fluorosis: Fluorosis is severe waterborne disease caused by high concentration of fluoride in groundwater. It is endemic in at least 25 nations across the world.

Causative Agents: It is caused by excessive intake of fluorides from many sources in food, water, air (gaseous from industrial waste), and excessive use of toothpaste. But, drinking water is the most important source. Moderate-level chronic exposure is more usual. Acute high-level exposure to fluoride is rare owes to unintentional pollution of drinking-water or due to fires or explosions. Fluoride in water is mostly of geological origin. Water with high levels of fluoride is generally found at the base of high peaks and in regions where geographical deposits are amassed in sea. The ready-to-serve foods, beverages, and snacks with high content of black rock salt (CaF_2) have 157 ppm fluoride and red rock salts. Intake of some drugs, for instance, fluoro-quinolone antibiotics, few anti-depressants, anti-fungal drugs, cholesterol-lowering drugs, steroids and anti-inflammatory drugs, arthritis drugs, antacids, drugs for osteoporosis and otosclerosis contain fluoride and can lead to fluoride toxicity. The people with calcium deficiency or malnourished individuals are more susceptible to develop dental and skeletal fluorosis. Fluoride-rich foods, for instance, tea, ocean fish, gelatin, skin of chicken, fluoridated salt, and food with post-harvest fumigants and pesticides, act as source of fluoride.

The other environmental sources include cigarette smoke and industrial pollution, e.g. fluoride in dust and fumes from industries manufacturing steel, aluminium, enamel, pottery, glass, bricks, phosphate fertilizer, welding, refrigeration, rust removal, oil refining, plastics, drugs, toothpaste, chemicals, and automobiles. Diets rich in fat increase fluoride deposition in bones.

Manifestation of disease: Once the fluoride comes in the body through blood vessels in the mouth or through gastrointestinal route, it spreads in various organs and tissues in the body. Fluoride (F) being an electronegative element, having a negative charge, is attracted by positively charged ions like calcium (Ca^{++}). Bone and tooth having highest amount of calcium in the body, attract maximum fluoride and is deposited as calcium fluorapatite crystals. It is not essential that all signs manifest at the same time. The seriousness of disease depends on person's age, nutritional status, environment, renal function, quantity of fluoride consumed, genetic background, affinity to allergies, and factors, for example, hardness of the water due to presence of calcium and magnesium. The symptoms include:

Dental fluorosis: Staining and pitting of the teeth, damaged enamel.

Skeletal fluorosis: Stiffness and pain in joints and in severe cases, the bone structure may change and ligaments may calcify, with impairment of muscles and pain. Compression of vertebral canal and intervertebral foramen applies pressure on nerves, and blood vessels resulting in paralysis and pain. Effects of fluorosis on soft tissues/systems may result in:

- Abortions, still births, and children with birth defects are common
- Allergic manifestation like skin rashes
- Calcification of ligaments and blood vessel
- Fluoride can damage a foetus, if the mother consumes water/food with high concentrations of fluoride during pregnancy/breast feeding
- Muscle weakness & stiffness, pain in the muscle and loss of muscle power, incapability to undertake routine activities
- Nervousness and depression, tingling sensation in fingers and toes, excessive thirst and tendency to urinate

- Stomach-ache, excessive saliva, nausea, and vomiting after acute high-level exposure to fluoride, and
- Urinary tract manifestations including less urine with yellowish-red colour

Prophylactic measures: Fluorosis can be stopped by avoiding excessive intake of fluoride by individuals/community and its adverse effects can be reduced by:

- Alerting the public with information on fluorosis, importance of drinking safe water, and healthy diet for preventing and controlling fluorosis;
- Eradicating excessive fluoride from drinking water by chemical precipitation, Alum coagulation or flocculation, and electrolyte de-fluoridation, adsorption;
- Improving the nutritional status of population/individuals at risk;
- Removing excessive fluoride from drinking water;
- Using alternate water resources including, surface water, rainwater, and low fluoride ground water;
- Using alternative water sources;
- Using safe drinking water with safe fluoride levels;

A. **Bacterial Diseases**

Cholera: Cholera is an acute bacterial infection of the gastrointestinal tract and can lead to acute dehydration and death. Cholera is a global problem, particularly in emergency situations. It can be prevented by providing safe drinking water, sanitation and good hygiene.

Causative agents: Cholera is caused by bacterium *Vibrio cholera (V. cholera)*. The bacteria live in shallow, salty water on microscopic crustaceans. The bacteria also live as colonies of biofilms coating the surface of the water, plants, stones, shells, and similar items. Eggs of midges serve as a reservoir for cholera bacteria.

Manifestation of disease: Toxic strains of cholera bacteria produce a poison that causes violent diarrhoea in humans. Bacteria can rapidly cause severe epidemics.

Prophylactic measures: The provision of safe water, proper sanitation, and food safety are essential for stopping occurrence of cholera. Health education adopting preventive behaviour can avert contamination.

Diarrhoea: Diarrhoea is the main public health problem directly linked with water and sanitation, but providing suitable sanitation facilities can prevent waterborne diseases. Diarrhoea is caused by various microorganisms including viruses, bacteria, and protozoans. It results in loss of both water and electrolytes, which leads to dehydration and, in some cases, death. About four billion cases of diarrhoea per year results in 1.8 million deaths, over 90 percent of them are among children under five years of age. Frequent episodes of diarrhoeal disease make children more susceptible to other diseases and undernourishment.

Causative agents: Diarrhoea can be caused by different agents, the common being the bacteria such as Salmonella and Vibrio parahaemolyticus, and viruses such as norovirus, rotavirus, sapovirus, and astrovirus. Less common causal organisms include the bacteria causing bacillary dysentery, cholera, and Shiga toxin-producing *E. coli* infection.

Manifestation of disease: The disease manifests with sudden onset of recurrent loose or watery stools with vomiting and fever. Acute diarrhoeal diseases are generally communicated by contaminated hands or ingestion of contaminated food or drinks. The incubation period generally lasts from few hours to five days after exposure for bacterial diarrhoea and one to three days for viral diarrhoea. Acute diarrhoea can be managed by fluid and electrolyte replacement.

Prophylactic measures: The main protective measures include:

- Buying fresh food from hygienic and reliable sources;
- Cooking food thoroughly before consumption, mainly seafood and shellfish;
- Cleaning and disinfecting toilet used by infected persons;
- Drinking boiled or bottled drinks from reliable sources
- Maintenance of personal hygiene including hand hygiene, especially before handling food or consumption, and after using toilet;
- Maintenance of good food hygiene by choosing safe raw materials, keeping hands and utensils clean;
- Maintaining good environmental hygiene, indoor ventilation, proper sanitary facilities and drainage system;
- Separating raw and cooked food, thorough cooking, and keeping food at safe temperature to prevent foodborne diseases;
- Washing and peeling fruit and avoiding consumption of raw vegetables;
- Washing hands with liquid soap and water.

B. Other Waterborne Diseases

Malaria: It is a serious disease caused by a parasite carried by the mosquitoes. Humans get infected by mosquito bite. Malaria is caused by the protozoan parasite *Plasmodium.* In humans malaria is caused by four different species of Plasmodium, viz. *P. falciparum, P. malariae, P. ovale* and *P. vivax*. Sometimes human beings become infected with Plasmodium species that usually infect animals, such as *P. knowlesi*. The malarial parasite is transferred by female Anopheles mosquitoes, which generally bite between dusk and dawn. Malaria is an acute febrile illness with incubation period of seven days or longer. The most severe form is caused by *P. falciparum*. Variable clinical manifestations include fever, headache, muscular pain and weakness, vomiting, cough, diarrhoea, and abdominal pain. In severe cases, it may result in organ failure, such as acute renal failure, pulmonary oedema, widespread seizures, and circulatory failure, followed by coma and death.

Typhoid: It is a bacterial infection caused by consumption of contaminated food or water. Symptoms are categorized by headaches, nausea, and loss of appetite. Every year, approximately 12 million people are affected by typhoid. Typhoid fever is an acute illness linked with fever caused by *Salmonella enterica* serotype *Typhi* bacteria. It is caused by *Salmonella paratyphi*, a related bacterium that generally causes a less serious sickness. The bacteria are found in water or food.

Manifestation of disease: The disease spreads through contaminated food and water or through close contact with infected person. Signs and symptoms generally include a high fever, headache, stomach ache, and either constipation or diarrhoea. Most people with typhoid fever feel better after starting antibiotic treatment. Signs and symptoms develop gradually, often manifesting in one to three weeks after exposure. One of the most serious complications of typhoid fever is intestinal bleeding or holes in the intestine, which may develop in the third week of illness.

Prophylactic measures: Setting-up of public health goals can help in prevention and control of typhoid fever. However, safe drinking water, improved sanitation, washing hands with hot, soapy water and washing hands before eating or preparing food and after using toilet, avoiding consumption of raw fruits and vegetables can help in prevention of disease.

Schistosomiasis: Schistosomiasis is a disease caused by parasitic worms. At various stages of lifecycle, worms and their eggs live in freshwater snails, water, and human hosts. Swimming, bathing or washing in contaminated water, cause infection and can finally damage the liver, intestines, lungs, and bladder. Studies have shown that sufficient water supply and sanitation – which lessens contact with polluted surface water – can decrease the infection rates by 77 percent.

Trachoma: It is an eye infection that spreads mostly through poor hygiene is caused by lack of suitable water supplies and hazardous sanitation environments. About 6 million people are blind due to trachoma. It affects women two to three times more than men. Children are particularly vulnerable to its infection. Suitable water supplies can reduce infection rate by 25 percent.

Intestinal Worms: People get infected with intestinal parasitic worms by coming in contact with soil polluted with human faeces of an infected person, or by eating polluted food. Intestinal worms infect about 10 percent of people in the developing world and, depending upon the seriousness of the infection, lead to undernourishment, anaemia, or stunted growth. Children are mainly prone and usually have the largest number of worms. About 400 million school-age children are infected by roundworm, whipworm, and/or hookworm. Actually, roundworm and whipworm alone are likely to affect one-quarter of world's population. In addition to this, waterborne diseases are also caused by water-based recreational activities or drinking water contaminated by disease-causing microbes or pathogens. Some of the commonly recognized waterborne infections are:

Cryptosporidiosis (Cryptosporidium) Diarrhoeal disease

Causative Agent: Protozoan parasite *Cryptosporidium spp.*

The parasite passed in the excreta of an infected person or animal remains present in soil, food, water, or surface contaminated with the faeces is the most common cause of recreational water illness. Being resistant to chlorine with high survival time, it remains present in the environment. Mode of transmission includes accidental ingestion of oocytes, contact with domestic animal/livestock, consuming raw milk/contaminated foods/water, and contact with infected person.

Symptoms

Watery stools, stomach spasms, loss of appetite, weight loss, mild fever, and nausea

Incubation Period: Symptoms appear a week after exposure and persist for about two weeks

Prevention

- Properly washing hands with soap and water after toilet;
- By avoiding consumption of untreated water of water bodies during swimming;
- Proper hand washing after contact with domestic animals, pets, and their excreta;
- Avoiding contact with domestic animal; and
- Avoiding consumption of unpasteurized milk

Cyclosporiasis (*Cyclospora* spp.): Diarrhoeal illness

Causative Agent: *Cyclospora cayetanensis,* a protozoan parasite

Infection occurs after consuming contaminated food or water. The parasite remains in the environment for about 1 to 2 weeks after being passed in stool and causes infection in other person. It doesn't spread directly from one person to another. Cyclospora is more common in tropical and subtropical regions and its foodborne outbreak is linked to diverse types of fresh vegetables.

Symptoms

Watery diarrhoea, abdominal spasms, loss of appetite, weight loss and tiredness, fever, and vomiting

Incubation Period: Symptoms appear one week after exposure and can last for a few days to months.

Prevention

- Properly washing hands with soap and water after toilet;
- By avoiding consumption of food or water contaminated with the parasite;
- Washing of vegetables;
- Taking precautions while traveling to tropical and subtropical regions;
- Avoiding tap water, fountain drinks, ice, and raw eatables

Escherichia coli Infection (*E. coli* O157:H7)

Causative Agent: *E. coli* O157:H7 is one of hundreds of strains of the bacterium which can cause severe illness

Its infection is linked with eating undercooked contaminated ground beef, vegetables contaminated with cattle faecal matter, person-to-person contact in families and childcare centres is also common. Infection can also occur after drinking raw milk or drinking water contaminated by farm animals during swimming.

Symptoms: Severe bloody diarrhoea, abdominal cramps, mild fever, other symptoms may include non-bloody diarrhoea or no symptoms at all.

Incubation Period: Symptoms appear two to five days after infection and illness generally resolves in five to ten days.

Prevention

Taking proper hygiene and sanitation measures

Giardiasis: A diarrhoeal illness

Causative Agent: *Giardia intestinalis*, a single-celled, microscopic protozoan parasite

The parasite passed in the stool of an infected person or animal is protected by an outer shell which helps in its survival for long time and its infection occurs after accidental ingestion of parasite swimming or drinking or consuming contaminated foods. Giardia may be found in soil, food, water, or surfaces that have been contaminated with the faecal matter of humans or animals.

Symptoms

Diarrhoea, fatty floating faeces, gas and bloating, abdominal spasms, weight loss, and mild fever

Incubation Period: Symptoms generally appear 1 to 3 weeks after exposure and last for 2 to 6 weeks in healthy persons.

Prevention

- Washing hands after using the bathroom and before consuming food;

- Avoiding consumption of water while swimming;
- Avoiding consuming untreated water from water streams;

Harmful Algal Blooms (HABs)

Harmful algal blooms (HABs) or the blue-green algal blooms containing toxins cause illness in humans and animals

Causative Agent: Blue-green algae

Transmission occurs after exposure to scums or water containing high levels of microcystin and cyanotoxins which are accidentally swallowed while consuming contaminated water or fish or during recreational activities. It may also appear after inhaling airborne droplets containing toxins.

Symptoms

Rash/blisters, cough, breathless, congestion, sore throat, earache/eye irritation, diarrhoea, nausea

Incubation Period: Symptoms appear between hours to two days after exposure to the toxins and illness lasts for a few days

Hot Tub Rash or *Pseudomonas* Dermatitis/Folliculitis

Causative Agent: *Pseudomonas aeruginosa*

The disease is caused when a person comes in contact with contaminated water for a long duration. *Pseudomonas aeruginosa* is present in the environment, viz. water, and soil, and being microscopic, it can't be seen with a naked eye. Hot tub rash can affect people of all ages. Most rashes clear up in a few days without medical treatment. However, if your rash lasts longer than a few days, consult your healthcare provider.

Incubation Period: Symptoms of hot tub rash appear within a few days of swimming in a poorly maintained pool or contaminated lake or poorly maintained hot tub

Symptoms

Itchy spots on the skin which may turn bumpy red rash, pus-filled blisters around hair follicles

Prevention

- Proper cleaning of swimsuit and shower with soap after swimming
- Disinfecting water bodies and regular check of pH levels of hot tubs and pools

Legionellosis (*Legionella*) and Pontiac fever

Causative Agent: Exposure to the *Legionella* bacteria, *Legionella pneumophila.*

Legionnaires' disease is spread by water droplets in the air containing Legionella bacteria. Pontiac fever is a mild form of Legionnaires' disease with flu-like symptoms, while Legionnaires' disease is a lung infection caused by the bacteria *Legionella pneumophila.* The bacteria are found in water.

Symptoms

Muscle aches, headache, tiredness, loss of appetite, and cough, followed by high fever (102–105°F), pneumonia, and infrequent abdominal pain and diarrhoea. People get sick after inhalation of water droplets containing bacteria. Exposure can occur at home, workplace, hospitals, or other public places. Legionella organism is found in water systems and reproduce, like certain plumbing systems, hot water tanks, cooling towers, large air conditioning systems, and hot tubs. It doesn't spread from person to person.

Swimmer's Ear (*Otitis Externa*)

Causative Agent: Streptococcus, Staphylococcus, or Pseudomonas types of bacteria

Ear infection is caused by contaminated water left in ear after swimming. It is known as '*swimmer's ear*' or *otitis externa.* The infection occurs in the outer ear canal and causes pain and discomfort. Swimmer's ear is more common in children.

Symptoms

Itchiness in the ear, redness, and swelling, pain in infected ear followed by pus draining from the infected ear. The disease cannot spread from one person to another. Tingling, burning, or itching of the skin, small reddish pimples, small blisters, within minutes to days after swimming in contaminated water. Pimples may change into small blisters. Scratching the areas may result in secondary bacterial infections.

Prevention

- Keep ears as dry as possible
- Using a bathing cap and ear plugs, during swimming
- Drying ears after swimming or showering

8.5.2 Water-Washed Diseases

Water-washed diseases are those that occur because of non-availability of sufficient water for maintaining personal hygiene, including:

- Cleaning teeth
- Hand cleansing before preparation and/or food consumption
- Regularly cleaning the body
- Washing hair with soap or shampoo at least once a week
- Washing hands with soap, and ash, after using the toilet

Water-washed diseases are at times called '*water-scarce*' diseases since there is a problem if water supply is insufficient. They include:

- Fungal skin diseases, for example, ringworm
- Ophthalmic (eye) diseases, for example, trachoma and conjunctivitis
- Infections caused or carried by lice, mites, fleas, or ticks, for example, scabies (caused by mites) and louse-borne epidemic typhus

8.5.3 Water-Based Diseases

Water-based diseases are caused by parasites which spend a part of their lifecycle in water. Water-based diseases, for instance, bilharzia and dracunculiasis are caused by helminths. Dracunculiasis or guinea worm disease spread by drinking water contaminated with copepods that contain the larvae of the guinea worm. The guinea worm larvae enter water by emerging from skin of an infected person during washing or bathing. Efficient water treatment is required for preventing the incidence of disease. Water-related diseases spread by insects that propagate or feed in or near water bodies, for instance, malaria is spread by Anopheles mosquito. Water-related diseases are not linked with lack of access to clean drinking water or to hygiene and sanitation services, but the standing water provides a habitat for insects to breed. Other water-related diseases include onchocerciasis (spread by blackfly), dengue fever, and yellow fever (spread by mosquitoes).

8.5.4 Quality Dimensions of Water and Sanitation

Evaluation of water quality is one of the most important steps for achieving the quality dimensions. Many analytical methods are used to test for the presence of probable contaminants in a known volume of water and usually expressed as milligrams per liter, mg/l, or mg l^{-1}. A number of pathogenic microorganisms are present in water and the source of pathogens is human faecal matter. Hence, a number of tests have been devised to identify the faecal contamination due to pathogenic organisms. These tests can help in finding total coliforms, faecal coliforms, and *Escherichia coli* (*E. coli*). Coliforms are a group of bacteria found in human and animal faeces and soil. *'Total coliforms'* comprises of all bacteria belonging to this group. The presence of *'total coliforms'* shows the contamination of some kind; while the faecal coliforms are usually present in faeces. *E. coli* is generally found in the faeces of humans and warm-blooded animals. Presence of *E. coli* indicates faecal contamination and presence of pathogenic organisms.

A number of pathogens – such as *Giardia*, *Entamoeba histolytica* and some viruses survive in waters; thus, the existence of *E. coli* in water is a sign of contamination but its non-existence cannot declare that water is safe. Chemical contamination of water sources poses serious health problems. Presence of Fluoride in drinking water even in low concentration affects the teeth, lead to mottling of children's teeth but extreme exposure has harmful effects, like skeletal fluorosis, where fluoride accumulates in the bones causing stiffness and pain in joints and bones. Turbidity (cloudiness), colour, taste, and odour (smell), whether of natural or manmade origin, also affect water. Thus, drinking water must be free of tastes and odours. Colour in water is because of the presence of dissolved organic matter and metals for example iron and manganese. Colour can come from industrial pollution, for instance, dyes used in textile industry. Organic substances contribute to the odour in water. Thus, any change in the physical appearance of water can be significant. The other mitigation measures can be:

- Carbon sequestration
- Reuse and recycling of water
- Conserving wetlands to decrease the damage to water quality from storms
- Increasing green space
- Decreasing cemented surfaces to reduce runoff

Changing of climate and reduced food availability are resulting in desertification, and increasing the need for above-ground irrigation. Such schemes, if executed in areas where the incidence of waterborne parasitic diseases is more will have serious implications on human health. There are numerous ground-breaking methods, which can improve the water supply and sanitation, for instance:

- Demand-driven methods in rural water supply
- Community-led total sanitation
- Public–private alliances to ensure urban water supply
- Providing microfinance to women for improving access to water

The interventions, like proper health and hygiene, and maintenance of water quality standards can considerably contribute in decreasing the levels of diarrhoeal diseases. Interventions to improve water quality at household level can be more effective than those at the source. Unfortunately, in developing nations, public health concerns are generally raised on the institutional setting, such as municipal, hospitals, and environmental sanitation. The WHO strategies for drinking water quality stress on an integrated approach besides assessment of water quality and management from source. It emphasizes on quality protection and prevention of pollution and suggests practical and participatory approach to address the needs in developing nations.

BIBLIOGRAPHY

Bhatt, M. R. (1995) Women in water management: the need for local planning. Development Practice 5:254–258.

Bhattacharya, S. K. (2003) Progress in the prevention and control of diarrhoeal diseases since Independence. National Medical Journal of India 16:15–19.

Clasen, T., *et al.* (2006) Interventions to improve water quality for preventing diarrhoea. Cochrane Database of Systemic Reviews 3:782.

Davis, J., White, G., Damodaron, S. and Thorsten, R. (2008) Improving access to water supply and sanitation in urban India: microfinance for water and sanitation infrastructure development. Water Science and Technology 58:887–891.

Fewtrell, L. and Colford, J. M., Jr. (2005) Water, sanitation and hygiene in developing countries: interventions and diarrhoea--a review. Water Science and Technology 52:133–142.

Fewtrell, L., *et al.* (2005) Water, sanitation, and hygiene interventions to reduce diarrhoea in less developed countries: a systematic review and meta-analysis. Lancet Infectious Diseases 5:42–52.

Forstinus, N. O., Ikechukwu, N. E., Martins, P. E. and Ani, O. C. (2016) Water and waterborne diseases: A review. International Journal of Tropical Disease & Health 12(4):1–14.

Haller, L., Hutton, G. and Bartram, J. (2007) Estimating the costs and health benefits of water and sanitation improvements at global level. Journal of Water and Health 5:467–480.

Hernberg, S. (1992) Introduction to Occupational Epidemiology. Philadelphia: Lewis Publishers.

Hunter, P. R. (1997) Waterborne Disease: Epidemiology and Ecology. Hoboken, New Jersey: John Wiley & Sons, Inc.

Hutton, G., Haller. L. and Bartram, J. (2007) Global cost-benefit analysis of water supply and sanitation interventions. Journal of Water and Health 5:481–02.

Janine, M. H., Selendy, P. F. and Wafaie, F. (2019) Water and Sanitation-Related Diseases and the Changing Environment: Challenges, Interventions, and Preventive Measures. Hoboken, New Jersey: John Wiley & Sons, Inc.

Kumar, S. G. and Jayarama, S. (2009) Issues related to sanitation failure in India and future perspective. Indian Journal of Occupational and Environmental Medicine 13:104.

Kumar, S. G. and Kar, S. S. (2010) Sustainable behavioral change related to environmental sanitation in India: Issues and challenges. Indian Journal of Occupational and Environmental Medicine 14:107–108.

Levy, B. S. and Wegman, D. H. (1994) Occupational Health: Recognizing and Preventing Work-Related Disease. Boston: Little Brown.

Majra, J. P. and Gur, A. (2008) India needs a great sanitary awakening. Indian Journal of Occupational and Environmental Medicine 12:143.

Mara, D. and Horan, N. J. (2003) Handbook of Water and Wastewater Microbiology. London: Elsevier.

Nath, K. J. (2003) Home hygiene and environmental sanitation: a country situation analysis for India. International Journal of Environmental Health Research 13:19–28.

Pandve, H. T. (2008) Environmental sanitation: An ignored issue in India. Indian Journal of Occupational and Environmental Medicine 12:40.

Rosenstock, L. and Cullen, M. R. (1994) Textbook of Clinical Occupational and Environmental Medicine. Philadelphia: Saunders.

Sobsey, M. D. and Bartram, S. (2003) Water quality and health in the new millennium: the role of the World Health Organization Guidelines for Drinking-Water Quality. Forum of Nutrition 56:396–05.

VanDerslice, J. and Briscoe, J. (1995) Environmental interventions in developing countries: interactions and their implications. American Journal of Epidemiology 141:135–144.

WHO. (2003) Chromium in Drinking-Water. Geneva: World Health Organization.

WHO. (2011) Guidelines for Drinking-Water Quality. Geneva: World Health Organization.

9 Vector-Borne Diseases

"The truly healthy environment is not merely safe but stimulating"

—William H. Stewart

FACT FILE

As per the reports of WHO from 2015:

- Failure to effectively collect and dispose of solid waste increases the spread of disease-carrying vectors, for instance, rodents and insects.
- Vector-borne diseases account for more than 17 percent of all infectious diseases, causing more than 700,000 deaths annually.
- More than 3.9 billion people in over 128 countries are at risk of contracting dengue.
- Malaria causes more than 400,000 deaths every year worldwide, most of them children under 5 years of age.
- Diseases such as Chagas disease, Leishmaniasis, and Schistosomiasis affect hundreds of millions of people worldwide
- 893 million people in 49 countries globally remain susceptible to lymphatic filariasis and require preventive chemotherapy to stop the spreading of parasitic infection.
- Vector-borne diseases are preventable through informed protective measures.

9.1 INTRODUCTION

Vectors are living organisms that can spread infectious diseases between humans or from animals to humans. Many of these are blood sucking pests, which consume disease-producing microbes along with a blood meal from a diseased host and later inoculate it into a new host during their consequent blood meal. Vector-borne diseases are caused by parasites, viruses, and bacteria that are spread by mosquitoes, sand flies, bugs, blackflies, ticks, tsetse flies, mites, snails, and lice. Every year there are more than 700,000 deaths from diseases such as malaria, dengue, schistosomiasis, human African trypanosomiasis, leishmaniasis, chagas disease, yellow fever, Japanese encephalitis, and onchocerciasis, worldwide. The major vector-borne diseases, together, account for around 17 percent of all infectious diseases. The burden of diseases is maximum in the tropical and sub-tropical areas and they affect the poorest populations. The major outbreaks of dengue, malaria, chikungunya yellow fever, and Zika have troubled populations, claimed lives, and overwhelmed

DOI: 10.1201/9781003464785-9

health systems in many nations. Incidence of vector-borne diseases is governed by demographic, ecological, and social factors. Global trade, unplanned urbanization, and ecological challenges, for instance, climate change affect the spread of pathogen, making spreading season longer or causing diseases to occur in nations where they were earlier unidentified. Changes in farming practices due to difference in temperature and rainfall affect the spread of vector-borne diseases. The growth of urban slums, lacking reliable piped water or suitable solid waste management, renders the population in towns and cities at risk of viral and vector-borne diseases. Together, such factors influence the reach of vector populations and the transmission patterns of disease-causing pathogens. Mosquitoes are the best-known disease-causing vectors, other being the ticks, flies, sand flies, fleas, triatomine bugs, and freshwater aquatic snails.

9.2 TYPES OF VECTOR-BORNE DISEASES

9.2.1 Diseases Caused by Aedes

Chikungunya: Chikungunya is an infectious disease caused by the chikungunya virus. The virus is found in Africa, Southeast Asia, Indian subcontinent, and Indian Ocean islands. Human beings and primates are the natural hosts for the chikungunya virus.

Causative Agents: The virus spreads to humans by bite of an infected female *Aedes* species mosquito. These mosquitoes breed in or near human habitations and prefer to feed on humans in daylight, but may also bite in evening time.

Manifestation of Disease: Chikungunya infection is characterized by sudden onset of:

- Back pain
- Headache
- High fever
- Muscle pain
- Rash
- Severe joint pain mainly in the arms and legs

Most people feel better after seven to ten days though some people may develop long-term joint pain. The diagnosis is based on symptoms and established with a blood test. Incubation period is normally three to seven days with a range of 1 to 12 days. It cannot be spread directly from person to person. There is no specific treatment for the disease. The use of antipyretics and rest can provide relief for some symptoms.

Prophylactic Measures: Since no effective vaccine is available, the prevention from coming in contact with disease-carrying mosquitoes and controlling mosquito population can help in combating disease. Mosquito control can be achieved by using insecticides or biological control agents besides using mosquito repellents and wearing bite-proof long sleeves and trousers thus, personal protection and management of mosquitoes are important in inhibiting illness.

Dengue: Dengue fever is a mosquito-borne disease caused by dengue viruses and occurs in tropical and sub-tropical areas of the world.

Causative Agents: Only the female mosquito spreads the virus. The mosquito bites in the daytime, both inside and outside homes in containers holding water, and is more active after sunrise and before sunset. Other species of mosquito can transmit the virus but are not presently established in Australia. The mosquitoes breed in creeks, marshes, pools, or other water bodies.

Manifestation of Disease: The disease has a sudden onset and symptoms including:

- Bleeding, usually from the nose or gums
- Extreme headache and pain behind the eyes
- Fever for three to seven days
- Loss of appetite
- Muscle and joint pain
- Skin rash
- Vomiting and diarrhoea

Recovery is at times linked with prolonged weakness. Repeated episodes of dengue fever may result in extreme bleeding and shock but, with suitable treatment, are hardly serious. Diagnosis is done by clinical presentation and a blood test. Incubation period is 3 to 14 days, commonly four to seven days. After biting an infected person it takes 8 to 12 days before the mosquito can infect other people. The mosquito remains infectious for life. Dengue is not transmitted from person to person. No specific anti-viral treatment is available. The best options to treat the symptoms are acetaminophen or paracetamol.

Prophylactic Measures: There is no precise medicine for dengue. Early detection of progression and access to proper medical care lowers fatality rates.

Proximity of mosquito breeding sites to human inhabitation is an important risk factor for dengue. Presently, the key mode to control or prevent the transmission of dengue virus is to combat the mosquito by avoiding breeding of mosquito in and around houses, work place, schools, and healthcare facilities. Mosquitoes can be prevented from retrieving egg-laying surroundings by ecological management and modification. Breeding of mosquito can be achieved by properly disposing of solid waste and eradicating artificial man-made habitats, covering, emptying and washing of domestic water storage containers, and applying suitable insecticides on water storage containers. Using personal household protection methods, for example, window screens, repellents, insecticide cured materials, coils and vaporizers, and wearing clothing that minimizes skin exposure to mosquitoes is recommended.

Community engagement can be ensured by educating the community on the risks of mosquito-borne diseases and engaging community to improve participation and mobilization for sustained vector control. Emergency vector control measures, for instance, space spraying of insecticides during outbreaks may also be useful. Monitoring and surveillance of vector and species composition must be carried out to regulate the efficiency of control interventions.

Lymphatic Filariasis: The disease impairs the lymphatic system and results in irregular enlargement of body parts, causing pain, severe disability, and social stigma.

Causative Agents: Lymphatic filariasis is caused by infection of parasites categorized as nematodes (roundworms). There are three types of thread-like filarial worms:

- *Brugia malayi*
- *Brugia timori*
- *Wuchereria bancrofti* (responsible for 90 percent of the cases)

Adult worms nest in the lymphatic vessels and disturb the normal function of the lymphatic system. The worms can live for about 6–8 years and, during their lifetime, produce millions of microfilariae (immature larvae) that circulate in the blood. Mosquitoes are infected with microfilariae by feeding blood when biting an infested host. Microfilariae mature into infective larvae within the mosquito. When infected mosquitoes bite people, mature parasite larvae are left on the skin from where they can enter the body. The larvae then travel to the lymphatic vessels where they develop into adult worms, thus continuing a cycle of transmission. Lymphatic filariasis is transmitted by different types of mosquitoes, for example, by Culex mosquito, widespread across urban and semi-urban areas, Anopheles, found in rural areas, and Aedes.

Manifestation of Disease: Filariasis infection is asymptomatic, acute, and chronic conditions, with no external signs of infection but damages the lymphatic system and kidneys, and changes body's immune system. At chronic stage it results in lymphoedema (tissue swelling) or elephantiasis (skin/tissue thickening) of limbs and hydrocele (scrotal swelling). Involvement of breasts and genital organs is common. Acute episodes of local irritation including skin, lymph nodes, and lymphatic vessels frequently accompany chronic lymphoedema or elephantiasis.

Prophylactic Measures: Mosquito control is the only approach used to minimize the spreading of lymphatic filariasis and other mosquito-borne infections. Depending on the parasite-vector species, methods, such as insecticide-treated nets, indoor residual spraying or personal protection measures may safeguard people from infection. The use of insecticide-treated nets in areas where *Anopheles* is the primary vector for filariasis improves the impact on transmission.

Rift Valley Fever: It is a viral zoonosis that mainly affects animals and human beings. The majority of human infections are due to contact with the blood or organs of infected animals. Human infections are due to bite of infected mosquitoes. So far, no human-to-human transmission of Rift Valley Fever (RVF) virus has been documented. Its incubation period varies from two to six days.

Causative Agents: RVF virus is a member of the *Phlebovirus* genus. The virus was first identified in 1931 among sheep in the Rift Valley of Kenya. The majority of infections in human beings are due to direct or indirect contact with blood or organs of infected animals. The virus can spread to humans during the handling of animal tissue while slaughtering, undertaking veterinary procedures, or disposal of carcasses. Herders, agrarian communities, slaughterhouse employees, and veterinarians are at high risk of infection. The virus infects human beings through inoculation, for instance, via a wound from an infested blade or through contact with cracked skin, or through breathing of aerosols produced during the slaughter of infected animals.

Manifestation of Disease: In mild form of disease, the incubation period varies from two to six days. Feverish syndrome with sudden onset of flu-like fever, muscle pain, joint pain, and headache are common symptoms. Some people may develop neck stiffness, sensitivity to light, loss of appetite, and vomiting. The symptoms generally last from four to seven days, after which the immune response becomes noticeable. While most cases are comparatively mild, a small percentage of patients may develop severe form of disease. This usually appears as distinct syndromes: ocular (eye) disease, meningoencephalitis, or haemorrhagic fever.

Prophylactic Measures: Outbreaks of Rift Valley Fever in animals can be stopped by a continuous programme of animal vaccination. Animal immunization must be executed before an outbreak if an epizootic is to be prevented. Once an outbreak has occurred, animal vaccination should not be executed because there is a threat of increasing the outbreak. Restricting or prohibiting the movement of livestock may be effective in slowing the spreading of the virus from infected to uninfected areas.

During an outbreak of RVF, close contact with animals, mainly with their body fluids, either directly or via aerosols, has been recognized as the most important risk factor for RVF virus infection. Awareness generation about the risk factors of RVF infection and individual protective measures can avoid mosquito bites. Public health communications for risk reduction should focus on decreasing the risk of animal-to-human spreading because of unsafe animal husbandry and slaughtering practices. Maintaining hand hygiene, wearing gloves, and other suitable specific protective equipment while managing sick animals can prove to be beneficial. In the epizootic regions, all animal products should be properly cooked before eating. Vector control measures at breeding sites are more effective if the breeding sites can be identified and are limited in size and extent.

Yellow Fever: It is a haemorrhagic condition resulting in high fever, bleeding, and cell death in liver and kidneys. If sufficient liver cells die, liver damages leading to jaundice. Mosquitoes spread yellow fever and can affect monkeys and humans. Yellow fever can occur in settlements close to the jungle, where infected monkeys and mosquitoes.

Causative Agents: Yellow fever is an acute viral haemorrhagic disease spread by infected mosquitoes. The "yellow" refers to jaundice that affects some patients. The virus causing yellow fever is an arbo-virus and is spread by mosquitoes, belonging to the *Aedes* and *Haemogogus* species.

Manifestation of Disease: Initially, the people with yellow fever don't develop symptoms, or the symptoms are very mild. Its incubation period is between three and six days. The disease cannot spread among humans. Only mosquitoes spread disease among humans. In the early acute stage, the individual may experience:

- Chills
- Dizziness
- Headache
- High grade fever
- Loss of appetite
- Nausea
- Painful muscles, mainly the back and knee muscles
- Vomiting

These symptoms generally last for seven to ten days. It's difficult to diagnose the disease, mainly during the early stages. It is often confused with severe malaria, leptospirosis, viral hepatitis, other haemorrhagic fevers, infection dengue fever, and poisoning. Polymerase Chain Reaction testing in blood and urine can help in detection of the virus in the early stages of the disease. In later stages, testing to detect antibodies is needed. The mosquito lives in different habitats and some breed around houses and others in the forest. There are three types of transmission cycles:

Sylvatic Yellow Fever: In tropical rainforests, monkeys, the main reservoir of yellow fever, are bitten by wild mosquitoes, which spread the virus to other monkeys. Sometimes the humans working or travelling in the forest are bitten by infected mosquitoes and develop yellow fever.

Intermediate Yellow Fever: In this type of spreading, semi-domestic mosquitoes infect both monkeys and people. The contact between people and infected mosquitoes results in increased transmission.

Urban Yellow Fever: Large epidemics occur when infested people transfer the virus into thickly populated areas with high density of mosquitoes and where most people lack immunity, due to lack of vaccination. In these circumstances, infected mosquitoes spread virus from person to person.

Prophylactic Measures: Vaccination is the main method of preventing yellow fever. The vaccine is safe and inexpensive and a single dose offers life-long protection against the disease. A booster dose of yellow fever vaccine is not required. Some of the vaccination strategies used to prevent yellow fever disease and transmission are:

- Mass vaccination campaigns to increase coverage in nations at risk
- Routine infant immunization
- Vaccination of people visiting the endemic areas

People generally excluded from vaccination include:

- Infants below nine months
- People allergic to egg protein
- People with severe immunodeficiency, and
- Pregnant women

The risk of spreading of yellow fever can be abridged by eradicating probable mosquito breeding sites and applying larvicides to water storage containers. Rapid detection of yellow fever and quick response through emergency vaccination campaigns are vital for regulating the outbreaks.

Zika: The disease is caused by a virus transmitted by Aedes mosquito, which bites during the daytime.

Causative Agents: Zika virus, a mosquito-borne flavivirus, the causative agent was first detected in Uganda in monkeys in 1947. Outbreaks of Zika disease have been recorded in Africa, America, Asia, and Pacific. From the 1960s to 1980s, rare cases of human infections were found across Africa and Asia, usually complemented by mild illness.

Manifestation of Disease: The incubation period of Zika virus disease is 3–14 days. Most of the people infected with Zika virus do not develop symptoms. Symptoms are usually mild including fever, rash, conjunctivitis, muscle and joint pain, sickness, and headache and generally last for two to seven days. Zika virus infection during pregnancy causes microcephaly and other hereditary deformities in the developing foetus and newborn. Zika infection in pregnancy leads to fatal loss, stillbirth, and pre-term birth. Zika virus is mainly spread by the bite of an infected mosquito from *Aedes* genus, mostly *Aedes aegypti*, in tropical and sub-tropical regions. *Aedes* mosquitoes generally bite during the day. The virus is also transmitted from mother to foetus during pregnancy, through sexual contact, blood transfusion, and organ transplantation. Diagnosis can only be established through laboratory tests of blood or other body fluids. No treatment is available for Zika virus infection or linked diseases. Symptoms of Zika virus infection are generally mild. The symptoms are fever and rash.

Prophylactic Measures: Protection against mosquito bites is a key prophylactic measure to prevent Zika virus infection. Special care should be taken to avoid mosquito bites mainly the pregnant women, women of reproductive age, and young children. Personal protection measures include wearing clothes covering most of the body; using physical barriers and applying insect repellent to skin or clothing. It is important to remove mosquito breeding sites, including:

- Cleaning up trash and used tires
- Covering water containers
- Eradicating standing water in pots

Community schemes to support local government and public health programmes reduce mosquito breeding sites. No vaccine is yet available for prevention or treatment of Zika virus infection. Zika virus can spread through sexual intercourse. Pregnant women must practice safer sex or abstain from sexual activity for at least entire duration of pregnancy.

9.2.2 Diseases Caused by Anopheles

Malaria: Malaria is distributed worldwide throughout the tropics and sub-tropics.

Causative Agents: Malaria is caused by protozoa of the genus *Plasmodium.* Four species cause disease in humans, viz. *Plasmodium falciparum, Plasmodium vivax, Plasmodium ovale,* and *Plasmodium malariae.* Other species of plasmodia infect reptiles, birds, and other mammals. Malaria is spread to humans by the bite of female mosquitoes of the genus *Anopheles.*

Manifestation of Disease: The symptoms of malaria are:

- Abdominal Pain
- Anaemia
- Bloody stools
- Cough
- Chills
- Convulsions
- Coma
- Nausea, vomiting, and diarrhoea
- Excessive sweating
- High fever
- Headache
- Muscle pain

Diagnosis: Identification of plasmodia in blood smears helps in the diagnosis of Malaria and treatment involves the use of quinine, quinidine, and pyrimethamine.

Prophylactic Measures: Chemoprophylaxis and personal shielding methods against mosquito vector and community-based methods help in regulating the vector. Exposure to *Anopheles* mosquitoes can be reduced by using protective repellents, insecticides, and bed nets.

9.2.3 Diseases Caused by Culex

Japanese Encephalitis: The disease was reported for the first time in 1871 in Japan. In temperate regions of Asia, Japanese encephalitis spreads during warm season. In tropics and sub-tropics, spread of disease rises during the rainy season.

Causative Agents: The disease is caused by virus Japanese encephalitis, the mosquito-borne flavi-virus. Japanese encephalitis spreads through bite of infected mosquitoes of *Culex* species. The virus exists in a transmission cycle between mosquitoes, pigs, and/or water birds. The disease is mostly common in rural and sub-urban settings, where humans live closer to vertebrate hosts.

Manifestation of Disease: Most infections are moderate with malaise and headache or without clear symptoms and the incubation period is between 4-14 days. In children, abdominal pain and vomiting are the initial symptoms. Severe disease is characterized by high fever, headache, rigidity in neck, confusion, coma, seizures, paralysis, and finally the death. A laboratory test confirms Japanese encephalitis infection. There is no antiviral for Japanese encephalitis but involves supportive treatment to relieve symptoms.

Prophylactic Measures: The prevention and control activities include immunization, and better-quality surveillance and reporting systems. To reduce the risk for Japanese encephalitis precautions must be taken to avoid mosquito bites. Personal preventive measures include the use of repellents, long-sleeved clothes, coils, and vaporizers.

9.2.4 Diseases Caused by Sand Flies

Leishmaniasis: The disease is caused by pathogenic protozoan parasite of genus Leishmania. Infection starts when a sand fly vector inoculates *Leishmania* parasites in the skin of a mammalian host. *Leishmania* causes a variety of inflammatory cutaneous disease.

Causative Agents: Leishmaniasis starts with a bite of female sand fly vector. Protozoa are inoculated into mammalian skin during a sand fly blood meal. The most common type of leishmaniasis is cutaneous leishmaniasis, when the parasites remain localized in skin tissue and leads to skin ulcers, which can self-heal without treatment.

Manifestation of Disease: The disease manifests as:

Cutaneous Leishmaniasis: With ulcers in skin

Mucocutaneous Leishmaniasis: Is rare form of the disease, caused by the cutaneous form of parasite and occurs once the skin ulcers heal. In this leishmaniasis, the parasites spread to nose, throat, and mouth.

Visceral Leishmaniasis: Known as systemic leishmaniasis or kala azar occurs two to eight months after bite of sand fly and damages internal organs, for instance, spleen and liver. It also affects bone marrow, as well as immune system, and harms these organs. The disease is found everywhere in the world excluding Australia and Antarctica. Common signs and symptoms are:

- Bleeding
- Decreased production of blood cells
- Enlarged liver
- Enlarged spleen
- Fever that lasts for weeks or months
- Swollen lymph nodes
- Weakness
- Weight loss

Diagnosis of cutaneous leishmaniasis is done by biopsy of ulcers. Chemical stains of bone marrow can help identify immune cells infected with the parasite.

Prophylactic Measures: No vaccine is available but the only way to prevent leishmaniasis is avoiding the bite of a sand fly. Other measures are:

- Avoiding moving outdoor during dusk and dawn, when sand flies are most active
- Indoor spraying of insecticides in sleeping areas
- Using insect repellent
- Using a bed net
- Using indoor screens and air conditioning when possible
- Wearing clothes that cover most of skin

Sand-fly Fever: Sand fly fever viruses are endemic among humans in several regions of the world, including Asia, Europe, and other continents. The disease was first recognized among American soldiers. It is also known as 'three-day fever' and is the viral infection that results in self-limited influenza-like symptoms categorized by a rapid onset.

Causative Agents: Three types of Phelebo virus are known to cause the fever, viz. Naples virus, Sicilian virus, and Toscana virus. The disease occurs commonly during summers and mainly in August when the sand flies are active.

Manifestation of Disease: Patients generally experience high grade fever with backache, muscular pain, and photophobia, followed by weakness, low BP, and feeble pulse. The accompanying symptoms include loss of appetite, headache, diarrhoea, stomach-ache, nausea, vomiting, and pain behind the eyeball. The diagnosis is made by carrying out serologic tests. So far no vaccine is available but the patients become resistant for two years against sand fly fever.

Prophylactic Measures: Avoidance of sand fly bites, control of sand flies, and breeding areas with insecticides are main methods for prevention.

9.2.5 Diseases Caused by Tse-Tse Flies

Sleeping Sickness: Sleeping sickness, known as African trypanosomiasis is a prevalent tropical disease, which can be fatal if not treated.

Causative Agents: It spreads by bite of an infected tse-tse fly with the flagellate protozoan *Trypanosoma brucei gambiense*, or the closely related subspecies *T. brucei rhodesiense*, a species native to the African continent.

Manifestation of Disease: The tse-tse fly bite explodes into a red sore and within few weeks the person experience fever, swollen lymph glands, aching muscles, and joints, headache and irritability. In progressive stage, the disease affects the central nervous system and alters the biological clock, resulting in confusion, unclear communication, seizures, and difficulty in moving. It involves two stages of illness, the first when the infected persons usually experience fever, headache, muscular and joint pain, and swelling of lymph nodes, followed by second stage, which develops within several weeks as in case of *T. brucei rhodesiense* or within one to two years as in case of *T. brucei gambiense*. It affects brain and spinal cord, with behavioural changes, insomnia, and intense fatigue, ending in death. The disease appears when *T. brucei* are transferred by tse-tse flies during the sucking of human blood. The flies get infected while feeding on blood of infected people or other infected mammals. Generally within 15 days after picking up the parasites, the flies become infective for humans. The trypanosomes multiply by binary division in the midgut of fly, and then travel to the salivary glands, and come out of fly's proboscis in drops of saliva during the bloodsucking. After an incubation period of one to two weeks, the trypanosomes are found in significant numbers in circulating blood, followed by invasion of lymph nodes and spleen, which becomes inflamed, soft, and tender, which is the main sign of disease. Erratic fever and deferred pain sensation are typical symptoms of disease. Microscopic examination of blood and lymph for presence of trypanosomes helps in diagnosing the disease which shows increased levels of WBCs.

Prophylactic Measures: The main approach of monitoring African trypanosomiasis is decreasing the reservoirs of infection and tse-tse fly. Screening of people at risk helps in categorizing the patients at an early stage. Regular screening of communities in tse-tse fly endemic areas and personal approaches, for instance, the use of insect repellent and wearing long-sleeved shirts and pants can reduce the incidence of sleeping sickness.

9.2.6 Diseases Caused by Fleas

Plague: Plague is caused by the zoonotic bacteria *Yersinia pestis*, usually found in small mammals and their fleas. It is transmitted by fleas from rats to humans. People infected with *Y. pestis* often develop symptoms after an incubation period of one to seven days.

Causative Agents: Humans get infected through the bite of infected vector fleas, unprotected contact with infectious body fluids or contaminated material, and inhaling respiratory droplets/small particles released by a patient with pneumonic plague.

Manifestation of Disease: There are two main clinical forms of plague: bubonic and pneumonic. Bubonic plague is the most common form and is characterized by painful swollen lymph nodes or 'buboes'. People infected with plague usually develop non-specific systemic symptoms after an incubation period of one to seven days, for instance, abrupt onset of fever, chills, head and body aches, weakness, vomiting, and nausea.

Bubonic plague is the most common form of plague and is caused by the bite of an infected flea. *Y. pestis* enters at the site and travels through the lymphatic system to the nearest lymph node where it replicates itself. The lymph node then becomes inflamed, tense, and painful, and is called a '*bubo*'. At progressive stages of infection, the swollen lymph nodes can turn into open sores filled with pus. Human to human transmission of bubonic plague is rare. Bubonic plague can advance and spread to the lungs and is known as pneumonic plague. Pneumonic plague is the most contagious form of plague. Incubation can be as short as 24 hours. Any person with pneumonic plague may spread the disease via droplets to other humans. Pneumonic plague, if not diagnosed and treated early can be fatal. Confirmation of plague requires laboratory testing. The best way is to identify *Y. pestis* in a sample of pus from a bubo, blood, or sputum. *Y. pestis* antigen can be detected by different techniques. Antibiotics and supportive therapy are effective against plague if diagnosis is made in time.

Prophylactic Measures: Preventive measures include counselling people when zoonotic plague is present in their environment and directing them to take precautions against flea bites and not to handle animal carcasses. People should be advised to avoid direct contact with infected body fluids and tissues. The plague outbreaks can be managed by:

- Developing environmental management programmes to understand the natural zoonosis of the disease cycle and to check spread
- Disinfection
- Ensuring accurate treatment
- Ensuring safe burial practices
- Finding and stopping the source of infection (including vector and rodent control)
- Isolating patients with pneumonic plague to reduce spread

- Protecting health workers by informing and training them on prevention and control
- Surveillance

9.2.7 Diseases Caused by Aquatic Snails

Schistosomiasis: The disease is common in people dealing with routine agricultural, household, work-related recreational activities, which expose them to infested water. Lack of hygiene and activities like swimming or fishing in infected water make them susceptible to infection.

Causative Agents: Schistosomiasis is caused by blood flukes of the genus *Schistosoma*.

Manifestation of Disease: People develop infection when the larva of parasite, released by freshwater snails enters the skin during the contact with infested water. Transmission occurs when diseased people contaminate water sources with excreta containing eggs, which hatch in water. The larvae, after entering the body develop into adult schistosomes, which live in the blood vessels where the female lays eggs. Some eggs pass out of the body in faeces or urine and continue parasite's lifecycle, while others become trapped in body tissues, causing immune reactions and damaging organs. Intestinal schistosomiasis causes abdominal pain, diarrhoea, and blood in the stool. Liver enlargement is common in advanced cases, and is often linked with accumulation of fluid in peritoneal cavity which leads to enlargement of spleen.

The sign of urogenital schistosomiasis is haematuria (blood in urine) and fibrosis of bladder and ureter in advanced cases. In women, urogenital schistosomiasis cause genital lesions, vaginal bleeding, and nodules in the vulva, while in men, urogenital schistosomiasis induces pathology of seminal vesicles, prostate, and other organs. In children, schistosomiasis can cause anaemia, stunted growth, and reduced ability to learn. Chronic schistosomiasis can result in death.

Schistosomiasis is diagnosed through the finding of parasite eggs in stool or urine specimens. Antibodies and/or antigens in blood or urine samples also indicate infection. Praziquantel is the recommended for treatment against all forms of schistosomiasis. It is safe and cost-effective drug.

Prophylactic Measures: Control of schistosomiasis can be ensured by:

- Access to safe water
- Improved sanitation
- Hygiene education
- Snail control

9.2.8 Diseases Caused by Lice

Typhus/Louse-borne Relapsing Fever: The disease is caused by infection with one or more rickettsial bacteria.

Causative Agents: There are three different types of typhus, and each type is caused by a different bacterium and spread by a different type of arthropod. There are three different types of typhus:

- **Epidemic (Louse-Borne) Typhus:** Caused by *Rickettsia prowazekii* and carried by body louse
- **Endemic (Murine) Typhus:** Caused by *Rickettsia typhi* and is carried by the rat flea or cat flea
- **Scrub Typhus:** Caused by *Orientia tsutsugamushi* and carried by mites in their larval stage

The type of typhus depends on what bites a person. Typhus outbreaks generally occur in developing countries or in regions of poor sanitation. Untreated typhus can have serious repercussions, and it's possibly fatal. Typhus is not transmitted from person to person like a cold or the flu.

Manifestation of Disease: Fleas, mites, lice, or ticks transmit it during the bite. Once in the bloodstream, the bacteria continue to reproduce and grow. Symptoms differ slightly by the type of typhus, but there are symptoms that are linked with all types of typhus, such as chills, fever, headache, and rash. Symptoms of epidemic typhus include:

- Confusion
- Eye sensitivity
- High fever (Above 102.2°F)
- Lethargy
- Low BP
- Rash
- Severe headache
- Severe muscular pain

The symptoms of endemic typhus last for 10 to 12 days and include:

- Diarrhoea
- Dry cough
- Nausea and vomiting

Symptoms seen in people with scrub typhus include:

- Cough
- Rash
- Red lesion or sore on the skin
- Swollen lymph nodes
- Tiredness

The incubation period for the disease is 5 to 14 days and symptoms won't appear for up to 5 to 14 days after bite. Diagnosis of typhus is difficult because symptoms are common to other infectious diseases, like dengue, malaria, and brucellosis. Diagnostic tests for the presence of typhus can be done by skin biopsy, western blot, and immunofluorescence test. Antibiotics most commonly used to treat typhus is doxycycline, chloramphenicol, or ciprofloxacin

Prophylactic Measures: Recommendations for prevention include:

- Escaping roaming in regions where typhus exposure has occurred
- Controlling the rodent population
- Keeping suitable personal hygiene

In addition to above mentioned diseases, some diseases are caused by ticks, for instance, Crimean-Congo haemorrhagic fever, Lyme disease, Relapsing fever, Rickettsial diseases (spotted fever and Q fever), Tick-borne encephalitis, Tularaemia, etc., and by Triatomine bugs, for instance, Chagas disease (*American trypanosomiasis*).

The World Health Organization provides strategic plans for strengthening of vector control as an important method to avoid disease and outbreak. To achieve this, re-alignment of vector control programmes is essential, backed by improved technical capacity, better-quality infrastructure, strengthened monitoring and surveillance systems, and community mobilization. Eventually, these will upkeep execution of an inclusive approach to vector control that allows the accomplishment of disease-specific national and global goals and contribute to attainment of the Sustainable Development Goals and Universal Health Coverage. The WHO responds to vector-borne diseases by:

- capacity building on clinical supervision, diagnosis and vector control;
- offering evidence-based guidance for monitoring vectors and safeguarding people against infection;
- offering technical support to nations so that they can efficiently handle cases and epidemics;
- supporting nations to improve their reporting systems; and
- sustaining the development and assessment of new tools, technologies, and methods for vector-borne diseases

A vital element in the management of vector-borne diseases is social change. Access to water and sanitation is a key factor in controlling and eliminating disease. The WHO works together with different government sectors to manage the vector-borne diseases.

BIBLIOGRAPHY

Alcais, A., Abel, L. and Casanova, J. L. (2009) Human genetics of infectious diseases: between proof of principle and paradigm. Journal of Clinical Investigation 119:2506–2514.

Brady, O. J., Smith, D. L., Scott, T. W. and Hay, S. I. (2015) Dengue disease outbreak definitions are implicitly variable. Epidemics 11:92–102.

Chala, B. and Feyissa H. (2021) Emerging and re-emerging vector-borne infectious diseases and the challenges for control: a review. Front Public Health 9:715–759.

Chu, K., *et al.* (1993) Parasitic Diseases in Water Resources Development: the Need for Intersectoral Negotiation. Geneva: World Health Organisation.

Gottdenker, N. L., Streicker, D. G., Faust, C. L. and Carroll, C. R. (2014) Anthropogenic land use change and infectious diseases: AReview of the Evidence. Ecohealth 11:619–632.

Gryseels, B., Polman, K, Clerinx, J and Kestens, L. (2006) Human schistosomiasis. Lancet 36(8):1106–1118.

Gubler, D. J. (2011) Dengue, urbanization and globalization: The unholy trinity of the 21st century. Tropical Medicine and Health 39:3–11.

Harvell, C. D., *et al.* (2002) Climate warming and disease risks for terrestrial and marine biota. Science 296:2158–2162.

Hassell, J. M., Begon, M., Ward, M. J. and Fèvre, E. M. (2017) Urbanization and disease emergence: Dynamics at the wildlife–livestock–human interface. Trends in Ecology and Evolution 32:55–67.

Hernberg, S. (1992) Introduction to Occupational Epidemiology. Philadelphia: Lewis Publishers.

Jones, B. A., *et al.* (2013) Zoonosis emergence linked to agricultural intensification and environmental change. Proceedings of the National Academy of Sciences of the United States of America 110:8399–8404.

Karesh, W. B. (2012) Ecology of zoonoses: Natural and unnatural histories. Lancet 380:1936–1945.

Kibret, S., *et al.* (2016) Malaria and large dams in sub-Saharan Africa: future impacts in a changing climate. Malaria Journal 15:448.

Kock, R. A. (2015) Vertebrate reservoirs and secondary epidemiological cycles of vector-borne diseases. Revue Scientifique et Technique 34:151–163.

Lafferty, K. D. (2009) The ecology of climate change and infectious diseases. Ecology 90:888–900.

Lashley, F. R. (2004) Emerging infectious disease: Vulnerabilities contributing factors and approaches, Expert Review of Anti Infective Therapy 2:299–316.

Levy, B. S. and Wegman, D. H. (1994) Occupational Health: Recognizing and Preventing Work-Related Disease. Boston: Little Brown.

McFarlane, R. A., Sleigh, A. C. and McMichael, A. J. (2013) Land-use change and emerging infectious disease on an island continent. International Journal of Environmental Research and Public Health 10:2699–2719.

Medlock, J. M. and Leach, S. A. (2015) Effect of climate change on vector-borne disease risk in the UK. Lancet Infectious Diseases 15:721–730.

Mellor P. S. and Leake, C. J. (2000) Climatic and geographic influences on arboviral infections and vectors. Revue Scientifique et Technique 19:41–54.

Nii-Trebi, N. I. (2017) Emerging and neglected infectious diseases: insights, advances, and challenges. Biomed Research International 5245021:1–15.

Ogden, N. H. and Lindsay, L. R. (2016) Effects of climate and climate change on vectors and vector-borne diseases: ticks are different. Trends Parasitol 32:646–656.

Rosenstock, L. and Cullen, M. R. (1994) Textbook of Clinical Occupational and Environmental Medicine. Philadelphia: Saunders.

Savi, S., *et al.* (2014) Emerging vector-borne diseases incidence through vectors. Front Public Health 2:267.

Simpson, D. I. (1964) Zika virus infection in man. Royal Society of Tropical Medicine and Hygiene 58:335–338.

Siraj, A. S., *et al.* (2014) Altitudinal changes in malaria incidence in highlands of Ethiopia and Colombia. Science 343:1154–1158.

Swei, A., *et al.* (2020) Patterns, drivers, and challenges of vector-borne disease emergence. Vector Borne and Zoonotic Disease 20:159–170.

Tong, M. X., *et al.* (2015) Infectious diseases, urbanization and climate change: Challenges in future China. International Journal of Environmental Research and Public Health 12:11025–11036.

Vasconcelos, P. F. and Monath, T. P. (2016) Yellow fever remains a potential threat to public health. Vector Borne and Zoonotic Diseases 16:566–567.

Weaver, S. C. and Reisen, W. K. (2010) Present and future arboviral threats. Antiviral Research 85:328–345.

Weiss, R. A. and McMichael, A. J. (2004) Social and environmental risk factors in the emergence of infectious diseases. Nature Medicine 10:70–76.

WHO. (2013) Vaccines and vaccination against yellow fever. Weekly Epidemiology Record 88:269–283.

WHO. (2017) World Malaria Report. Geneva: World Health Organization.

WHO. (2020) Vector-Borne Diseases. www.who.int/news-room/fact-sheets/detail/vector-borne diseases.

Wilder-Smith, A. and Gubler, D. J. (2008) Geographic expansion of dengue: The impact of international travel. Medical Clinics of North America 92:1337–1390.

Wilson, A. L., *et al.* (2020) The importance of vector control for the control and elimination of vector-borne diseases. PLOS Neglected Tropical Disease 14:e0007831.

10 Airborne Diseases

"Environmental pollution is not only humanity's treason to humanity but also treason to all other living creatures on earth!"

—Mehmet Murat Ildan

FACT FILE

- 99 percent of the world's population live in places where air pollution levels exceed WHO guideline limits
- An estimated 4.2 million deaths globally are linked to ambient air pollution, mainly from heart disease, stroke, chronic obstructive pulmonary disease, lung cancer, and acute respiratory infections

Worldwide ambient air pollution accounts for:

- 29 percent of deaths and disease from lung cancer
- 43 percent of deaths and disease from chronic obstructive pulmonary disease
- 25 percent of deaths and disease from ischaemic heart disease
- 24 percent of deaths from stroke
- 17 percent of deaths and disease from acute lower respiratory infection
- 29 percent of deaths and disease from lung cancer

10.1 INTRODUCTION

Air pollution is a major concern of new civilized world, which has a serious toxicological impact on human health and environment. It has a number of different emission sources, but motor vehicles and industrial processes contribute to a major part of air pollution. According to the World Health Organization, the six major air pollutants are particle pollution, ground-level ozone, carbon monoxide, sulphur oxides, nitrogen oxides, and lead. Long and short-term exposure to air suspended toxicants has a different toxicological impact on human including respiratory and cardiovascular (CV) diseases, neuropsychiatric complications, irritation in eyes, skin diseases, and long-term chronic diseases such as cancer. Several reports have revealed a direct association between exposure to poor air quality and increasing rate of morbidity and mortality mostly due to CV and respiratory diseases. Air pollution is considered as the major environmental risk in the incidence and progression of some diseases such as asthma, lung cancer, ventricular hypertrophy, Alzheimer's and Parkinson's diseases, psychological complications, autism, retinopathy, foetal growth, and low birth weight.

DOI: 10.1201/9781003464785-10

10.2 DEFINING AIR QUALITY

State of the air in the environment refers to '*Air quality*'. Good air quality refers to the air that is clean, clear, and free from pollutants, for instance, smoke, dust, and smog, among other pollutants in the air. Air quality is determined by measuring a range of pollution indicators. Good air quality is the basic requirement for maintaining the equilibrium of life on earth. In the absence of clean air, human health, plants, animals, and natural resources are exposed to air pollution. Poor air quality affects human health and/or the environment. Air quality is affected by natural or man-made causes which poses a threat to human health. Natural causes include volcanoes, wind, and dust storms. Man-made causes include emissions of toxic gases from vehicles, industries, thermal power plants, burning wood, or other material in open air or landfills. The term 'air quality' means:

"... the state of the air around us. Good air quality refers to clean, clear, unpolluted air. Clean air is essential to maintaining the delicate balance of life on this planet – not just for humans, but wildlife, vegetation, water and soil. Poor air quality is a result of a number of factors, including emissions from various sources, both natural and human-caused ..."

Day to day emissions from different air pollution sources degrade the air quality. The stationary sources includes power plants, manufacturing facilities, smelters, motor machines, and burning of fossil fuels; while mobile sources include vehicles; and natural sources include volcanic eruptions and windstorm dust. The pollutants from all sources released into the air affect human health and the environment. The quality of air depends on three factors:

- The extent of pollutants
- The rate at which the pollutants are released in the atmosphere
- Duration for which the pollutants are entrapped in an area

Air pollution releases a range of pollutants classified under different categories that include:

- Sulphur dioxide (SO_2)
- Particulate matter (PM)
- Hydrocarbons (HC)
- Volatile organic compounds (VOC)
- Lead
- Carbon dioxide (CO_2)
- Carbon monoxide (CO)
- Nitrogen oxides (NOx)
- Smog

Most of the air pollutants are gases, but some are tiny solid particles, like dust, smoke, or soot. Air pollution can also affect indoor air. Removing the pollutants from indoor air can improve the quality of indoor air. Indoor air pollutants include cigarette smoke, moulds, dust mites, formaldehyde, volatile organic compounds (VOCs), and radon gas. Air pollutants tend to remain in the air under certain conditions like light winds or mountains that curb the transference of pollutants away from an area.

10.2.1 Health and Air Quality

Air pollution with the presence of one or more contaminants in the atmosphere, such as dust, fumes, gas, mist, odour, smoke, or vapour, in large amounts and for a longer duration can harm human health. The respiratory tract is the main route of exposure to air pollution. Inhalation of air pollutants may lead to inflammation, oxidative stress, immunosuppression, and mutagenicity in cells, impacting the lungs, heart, brain among other organs, eventually leading to disease. Once the air pollutants enter the body, they circulate in the entire body through the bloodstream leading to systemic inflammation and carcinogenicity.

The specific health outcomes linked with exposure to air pollution include stroke, ischaemic heart disease, chronic obstructive pulmonary disease (COPD), lung cancer, pneumonia, and cataract. There is suggestive evidence linking air pollution exposure with increased risk of adverse pregnancy outcomes, which manifests in the form of low-birth weight, cancers, diabetes, cognitive impairment and neurological diseases. There are many adverse impacts of air pollutants on health, yet pollutants with strong evidence for public health concern include PM, carbon monoxide (CO), ozone (O_3), nitrogen dioxide (NO_2) and sulphur dioxide (SO_2). Fine PM is an important source of health risks, for these particles penetrate deep into the lungs, enter the bloodstream, and travel to organs resulting in systemic damage to tissues and cells. Both short- and long-term exposure to air pollutants can cause health problems in children and adults. The levels and duration of exposure that can be considered '*safe*' vary with the pollutant, as well as the related disease outcomes. Short-term exposure to high levels of PM can reduce the functioning of lungs, respiratory infections and aggravated asthma; while long-term or chronic exposure to fine PM increases the risk of non-communicable diseases including stroke, CV disease, COPD, and cancer. Children, elderly and pregnant women are more vulnerable to air pollution-related diseases. Heredity factors, comorbidities, nutritional factors and socio-demographic factors govern the susceptibility to air pollution. Maternal exposure to air pollution is linked with adverse birth outcomes. The health impacts from exposure to ambient air pollution or household air pollution depend on forms and concentration of pollutants in the air to which an individual is exposed. However, the health risks and disease pathways between ambient and household air pollution exposure are often similar, due to their comparable composition. The public health impacts of air pollution exposure range from increased hospitalization, to increased risk of premature death and disease. Air pollution can thus be categorized as:

Ambient Air Pollution: Presence of one or more substances in air at a concentration of, or for duration above the permissible levels with the possibility to produce adverse health impacts. The air pollution in the ambient environment is outdoor air, but it may enter homes.

Household Air Pollution: It refers to the air pollution produced by combustion of household fuel, resulting in indoor air pollution which can contribute to outdoor air pollution.

Almost the entire global population (99 percent) is exposed to air pollution levels that exceed the permissible limits for fine PM 2.5 $\mu g/m^3$, with low- and middle-income nations suffering from the maximum level of exposure.

10.2.2 Airborne Diseases

Air pollution is a major issue faced by the entire world. Both outdoor and indoor air pollution causes numerous health problems. The indoor air is five times more polluted than the outdoor air. In recent years, indoor air pollution has become a topmost cause of health issues in India. Pets, cooking smoke, household equipment, and electronic equipment are major sources of indoor pollution. The noxious particles enter the respiratory system through the nasal tract and cause respiratory problems. The increasing air pollution is necessitating the installation of air purifiers at household level to keep the indoor air safe and pollution free. The effects of air pollution result in common health impacts like irritation of eyes, nose, mouth and throat, headache and dizziness and respiratory and lung diseases, like:

- Asthma
- Birth defects and immunological defects
- CV disease and stroke
- Chronic obstructive pulmonary disease (COPD)
- Developmental deficits due to air pollutants, for instance, mercury
- Leukaemia (blood cancer linked with exposure to benzene vapours)
- Liver cancer (caused by inhalation of volatile carcinogenic chemicals)
- Lung cancer
- Mesothelioma (lung cancer linked with exposure to asbestos)
- Neurobehavioral/neurological problems
- Pneumonia
- Reduced lung function
- Premature death

According to the WHO, air pollution is linked to 7 million premature deaths.

Indoor Air Pollution

- 6 percent (Lung cancer)
- 12 percent (Acute lower respiratory infections in children)
- 22 percent (COPD)
- 26 percent (Coronary artery disease/ischaemic heart disease)
- 34 percent (Stroke)

Outdoor Air Pollution

- 3 percent (Acute lower respiratory infection in children)
- 6 percent (Lung cancer)
- 11 percent (COPD)
- 40 percent (Ischaemic heart disease)
- 40 percent (Stroke)

Airborne diseases pass from one person to another when microbes, for instance, bacteria, fungi, or viruses, move amidst air in aerosolized particles. These diseases can spread through cough or sneeze, spraying liquid, or dust. The microbes may come from a diseased person or animal or from soil, garbage, besides other sources. The infectious vehicles travel along air currents, stay in the air, or adhere to surfaces, where they are inhaled by someone else. Airborne transmission can occur over relatively long distances and spans of time. If you go into the bathroom that someone coughed in minutes before, it could be a danger. This makes it possible for airborne diseases to infect larger numbers of people and more difficult to determine the causes due to a lack of person-to-person contact. Airborne transmission has varying means. Airborne diseases can travel distances greater than six feet and remain infectious in the air from minutes to hours. This largely depends on the type of ventilation and preventative measures inside the building.

There are numerous airborne diseases, but the causes, symptoms, and treatment may vary. Prevention of transmission includes the use of personal protective equipment and operational ventilation system. Airborne diseases appear around the globe and virtually trouble everyone; however, the incidence is lower in the nations where vaccines are available and inexpensive.

Airborne diseases can spread through a direct or an indirect form of transmission, depending on the causative agent involved. The pathogens may enter the air in wet droplets, for example, during breathing or sneezing. They remain suspended in the air, and some droplets dry out, leaving aside the microscopic particles. The suspended particles attach to or enter the body of living organisms. Some microbes, like *Aspergillus*, are widely present in the environment, mainly in soil, plants, including decaying plant matter, household dust, and construction materials, besides food and water. During repair, breathing in dust containing fungus may cause disease. Likewise, anthrax, too, is present in the soil. A person becomes sick after inhaling dust containing anthrax spores.

Symptoms: Airborne diseases usually result in one or more of the following symptoms:

- Body aches
- Congestion
- Coughing
- Fatigue
- Fever
- Headache

- Inflammation of nose, throat, sinuses, or lungs
- Loss of appetite
- Runny nose
- Sneezing
- Sore throat
- Swollen glands

Many diseases spread through the air, including:

- Anthrax
- Aspergillosis
- Chickenpox
- Common cold
- Coronavirus and COVID-19
- Diphtheria
- Influenza
- Measles
- Meningitis
- Mumps
- Tuberculosis
- Whooping cough

10.2.3 Diseases Caused by Microbes

Besides air pollutants, airborne diseases are caused by pathogenic microbes. The microbes released by an infected person during coughing, sneezing, laughing, and close contact or release of aerosol containing microbes are harmful. The microbes once released remain in the air on dust particles and respiratory and water droplets, but their inhalation or contact of secretions with mucous membranes is enough for causing disease. Contact airborne diseases are transferred when an infected person comes in contact with an uninfected person and the microbe gets transmitted. These diseases can also be transferred by indirect contact with the environment of infected person or using the personal items. The body discharges or secretion increase the probable risk of spread and environmental contamination. Some of the airborne and direct contact diseases include:

Acute Flaccid Myelitis: It is a rare but severe neurologic condition that affects the spinal cord and results in the weakness of muscles and reflexes. The cause of AFM can be viruses, environmental toxins, and genetic disorders, listing poliovirus, non-polio entero-viruses, West Nile Virus, and adenoviruses among the potential reasons. The clinical manifestation includes fever, cough, vomiting, or diarrhoea. Weakness occurs in one or both limbs, and may go together with stiff neck, headache, or pain in the affected limbs. Staying away from mosquitoes that can transmit viruses and using products that repel mosquitoes can help in prevention. Following hand washing practices, using soap and water is good advice to prevent illness. Not sharing the food with an infected person and use of disinfectant to clean hard surfaces can also be beneficial.

Anthrax: It is a serious disease caused by *Bacillus anthracis*, a bacterium that produces spores. Anthrax usually occurs in wild or domesticated warm-blooded grazing animals for instance sheep and cattle, but can infect humans. Anthrax is a very rare disease, and generally occurs in farmers or people having close contact with animals or their products, particularly wool, animal hair, or skins. Infection involves skin, when the bacteria enter through a cut or abrasion. Infection can also occur if spores are inhaled or if the meat of an infected animal is consumed. Anthrax is a probable agent in biological warfare. Of the various forms of disease, cutaneous anthrax primarily involves skin, which then turns into a blister and then into a painless ulcer with a specific black region in the centre. There is generally marked inflammation around lymph glands. Inhalational anthrax may occur when spores are breathed in, which at first appears as flu-like illness, but afterwards results in severe breathing problems and shock. Lacking treatment, death generally occurs one to two days after the onset of severe symptoms. Intestinal anthrax may occur after consumption of contaminated meat. Symptoms may include nausea, loss of appetite, vomiting, fever, abdominal pain, vomiting of blood, and severe diarrhoea. Anthrax is generally diagnosed by isolating *Bacillus anthracis* from the blood, skin lesions, or respiratory secretions. The incubation period is usually one to seven days, but can be up to two months. Control of anthrax in livestock herds is important for prevention of its transfer to humans. Anthrax spores have been used in bioterrorist attacks in the United States of America.

Chickenpox: The disease also known as varicella is a highly contagious infection caused by the *Varicella zoster* virus. Although painful, most people improve within one to two weeks. Its incubation period is 10-21 days. It is highly contagious. The infection propagates in a similar way as colds and flu. A diagnosis can be done by observing the signs and symptoms. The itchy blister rash produced by infection appears 10 to 21 days after exposure to the virus and generally lasts for about five to ten days. Other signs and symptoms, before the rash, include fever, loss of appetite, headache, tiredness, and a general feeling of being unwell. Once the chickenpox rash appears, it goes through three phases, viz. raised pink or red papules, small fluid-filled vesicles, and crusts and scabs, which cover the broken blisters and take several days to heal. Chickenpox vaccine is effective in preventing the disease.

Enterovirus: *Enteroviruses* are a group of viruses of single-stranded RNA viruses linked with several human and mammalian diseases. *Enteroviruses* are named by their transmission route through the intestine and can cause a number of infectious illnesses which are generally mild. But if they infect the central nervous system, they can cause serious illness. The two most common ones are echovirus and coxsackievirus.

Group A Streptococcus – The Streptococcus bacterium is often found in throat and on skin. People carrying Group A streptococci have no symptoms of illness as these infections result in comparatively mild illnesses. Occasionally, these bacteria can cause severe and even life-threatening diseases.

Group B Streptococcus: Group B Streptococcus bacterium causes illness in newborn babies, pregnant women, elderly, and adults with illnesses, for instance, diabetes or liver disease. It is the most common life-threatening disease in newborns.

Influenza: It is caused by a virus and affects the nose, throat, and lungs and can cause life-threatening problems in many people.

Haemophilus Influenza: Disease caused by *Haemophilus influenzae* type B can affect many organ systems resulting in pneumonia, occult febrile bacteraemia, meningitis, epiglottitis, septic arthritis, cellulitis, otitis media, purulent pericarditis, and other less common infections, for instance, endocarditis, and osteomyelitis.

Measles: It is a respiratory disease caused by a virus that replicates in the nose and throat of an infected child or adult resulting in fever, runny nose, cough, and a rash all over the body. When infected person coughs, sneezes, or talks, droplets spray in the air, where other people inhale them. At times, the infected droplets may rest on a surface, where they remain active and contagious for several hours, which can act as a source of infection. Signs and symptoms of measles appear around 10 to 14 days after exposure to the virus; the important ones being fever, dry cough, runny nose, sore throat, inflamed eyes, skin rash, etc. The infection occurs in successive stages over a period of two to three weeks. Since measles is highly infectious after the rash breaks, people with measles must not interact with other people during this period. It is essential that non-immunized people be kept away from the infected person.

MRSA: Methicillin-resistant Staphylococcus Aureus is a bacterial infection which is resistant to some antibiotics. If MRSA bacteria are found on skin, these do not cause illness and result in pimples or boils.

Mumps: It is a contagious disease caused by a virus and usually starts with a few days of fever, headache, muscle ache, fatigue, and loss of appetite, followed by swelling of salivary glands, puffy cheeks, and a tender, swollen jaw. The virus passes from one person to another through saliva, nasal secretions, and close personal contact. The condition primarily affects the salivary glands and there may be complications like meningitis, pancreatitis, inflammation of the heart, permanent deafness, and testicular inflammation, which unusually results in infertility. No precise treatment is known. Efforts involve monitoring of symptoms with pain medication. Mumps is considered most contagious after the beginning of symptoms, and separation is suggested during this period.

Pertussis: Commonly known as whooping cough, is a respiratory disease which starts with flu-like symptoms that worsen after some days.

RSV: RSV is a virus that affects the lungs and respiratory tract. Healthy people generally experience mild, cold-like symptoms, but the virus can have serious implications for infants and older adults.

Smallpox: It is a serious and deadly viral infection, often communicable, meaning it spreads from person to person causing lasting scarring. At times, it causes deformity. Smallpox has affected the human race for thousands of years but was wiped out globally by 1980 after the discovery of the smallpox vaccine. It's no longer found in the world. An infected person can spread the virus through coughing or sneezing while talking.

Tuberculosis: A disease caused by a bacterium that usually attacks the lungs.

Varicella: A disease commonly known as chickenpox that is caused by a virus. The most common symptom is a skin rash found mostly on the face, scalp, and trunk.

Coronavirus and COVID-19: A fast spreading coronavirus, SARS-CoV-2, and the disease it causes, COVID-19, was accountable for millions of infections and hundreds of thousands of deaths worldwide in 2020. While the coronavirus that causes COVID-19 is usually not regarded as airborne, in some situations the virus acts like an airborne disease, for example, in clinical settings where people are receiving intensive medical treatment. In usual situations, SARS-CoV-2 spreads through cough or sneeze droplets, though the size of the droplets is larger than what is believed to be airborne. The common symptoms of COVID-19 include fever, cough, fatigue, and shortness of breath.

Common Cold: Millions of common cold cases occur each year. Usually, most adults get infected with it twice or thrice a year and children tend to get infected more frequently. Many viruses are responsible for cold, but it's generally a rhinovirus.

Influenza: Most people experience flu, which being contagious spreads easily before the appearance of first symptoms. The flu remains contagious for five to seven days. There are many strains of the flu, which constantly change making it difficult for the body to develop immunity.

Diphtheria: Once a major cause of sickness and death mainly among children, diphtheria is now a rare disease. It is a serious infection caused by a strain of bacteria called *Corynebacterium diphtheriae* that produces a toxin. Owing to widespread vaccination, fewer cases have been reported in the last few decades. The disease injures the respiratory system and damages the heart, kidneys, and nerves.

10.2.4 Health Implications of Air Pollution

Air pollution causes serious diseases related to lungs, heart, and brain, the important being:

Pneumonia: Pneumonia is often but not always due to infection. The infection may be bacterial, viral, fungal, or parasitic. It causes inflammation of air sacs in one or both lungs. Air sacs get filled with pus or fluid causing cough, fever, chills, and breathing.

Chronic Obstructive Pulmonary Disease (COPD): It is an inflammatory lung disease. In this, the flow of air in the lungs gets obstructed and also inhibits the breathing. Exposure to smoke, perfumed products, and exposure to products and paints intensify COPD. According to the World Health Organization, COPD causes approximately 25 percent of deaths in adults.

Lung Cancer: The carcinogen agents, $PM_{2.5}$ present in indoor air are linked with lung cancer. Indeed, air pollution causes nearly 17 percent premature deaths in adults. People working in congested areas or without ventilation are at risk of lung cancer.

Cardiovascular Problems: Both high arterial blood pressure and air pollution due to high levels of fine $PM_{2.5}$ have been linked with increased risks of CV diseases, including stroke, heart failure, and myocardial infarction. The air pollutants once inhaled travel deep into the bloodstream through the lungs, and reach the heart, thereby increasing the risk of developing heart and circulatory diseases. Air pollutants can damage the blood vessels by making them narrower and harder. Research has revealed that short- and long-term exposure to particulate pollution is linked with an increased risk of heart attacks and heart diseases.

In addition to the aforementioned diseases exposure to various toxic gases can have adverse health implications. Some of the health issues linked with these pollutant gases are discussed in the following pages.

Carbon-Monoxide Toxicity: Carbon monoxide produced as a result of combustion of fossil fuels, is basically a tasteless, odourless, colourless, and non-irritating gas. Its binding affinity to haemoglobin is much greater than oxygen and it forms carboxyhaemoglobin, consequently reducing oxygen-carrying capacity and utilization of oxygen. Hypoxia and toxicity can lead to cerebrovascular ischaemia and myocardial infarction. Carboxyhaemoglobin acts as a direct toxin at cellular level, and interrupts the cellular processes. It obstructs the aerobic metabolism, causing an inflammatory cascade that produces catastrophic damage to the CNS. Owing to both unintentional exposure and suicidal poisonings, acute toxicity of CO can be deadly, causing deaths.

The sources of CO in outdoor air are cars, trucks, and other vehicles or machinery that make use of fossil fuels. Various items, for instance, unvented kerosene, gas space heaters, leaking chimneys, furnaces, and gas stoves release CO which affects indoor air quality. Foetus, children, aged people, and people with anaemia or with a history of heart or respiratory disease probably experience more health issues when exposed to high levels of CO. Not only this, CO also contributes indirectly to climate change for it contributes in chemical reactions in the atmosphere that emit ozone, which is a climate change gas. Moreover, CO has a direct but a weak effect on climate. Consequently, CO is categorized as a short-lived climate forcing agent, triggering CO emission reductions to be considered as a possible strategy to ease impacts of global warming. It has been noticed that CO poisoning cases tend to increase during winters, which is most often related to increased level of indoor CO subsequent to the use of inappropriately vented space heaters and use of gas ranges to heat the house.

Sources: Sources of CO include:

- Auto, bus, or truck exhaust from garages, adjacent to roads, or parking areas
- Automobile exhaust from garages
- Furnaces, gas water heaters, wood stoves and fireplaces
- Damaged or poorly adjusted and retained combustion devices (e.g., boilers, furnaces)
- Gas stoves
- Generators and other gasoline-based equipment
- Improperly sized, blocked, or disconnected chimney
- Incomplete oxidation during combustion in gas ranges, and unvented gas or kerosene heaters
- Leaking chimney
- Leaking chimneys and furnaces
- Tobacco smoke
- Unvented kerosene and gas space heaters

Health Implications and Symptoms: At low concentrations, CO may result in:

- Tiredness in healthy people
- Chest pain in people with CV diseases

At moderate concentrations, it may lead to:

- Angina
- Impaired vision
- Reduced brain function

At higher concentrations, it may result in:

- Confusion
- Dizziness
- Flu-like symptoms that decrease after leaving home
- Headaches
- Impaired vision and coordination
- Nausea

At very high concentrations, CO may turn out to be fatal. Acute effects are due to the formation of carboxyhaemoglobin in the blood, which obstructs the oxygen carrying capacity of blood.

Aetiology and Pathophysiology: When haemoglobin is exposed to CO, carboxyhaemoglobin complex is formed within red blood cells, which is consequent of binding to haemoglobin with an affinity of 200 times that of oxygen. Methylene chloride, an industrial solvent and component of paint remover, when metabolized produces CO. A small amount of CO is generated endogenously with the breakdown of heme, and every person has a detectable amount of carboxyhaemoglobin at baseline. This is typically 1 to 3 percent in non-smokers and 10 to 15 percent in smokers. By substituting oxygen, CO decreases the oxygen-carrying capacity and oxygen delivery to tissues, causing marked cellular hypoxia and acidosis. CO directly upsets multiple metabolic processes. CO binds to mitochondrial cytochrome oxidase, directly preventing aerobic metabolism. CO fixes to cytochrome c oxidase in the brain, causing impaired mitochondrial function and ATP synthesis, platelet to neutrophil accumulation, and neutrophil degranulation. Myeloperoxidase, proteases, and reactive oxygen species are consequently liberated, causing cellular damage. In endothelial cells, proteases (via xanthine dehydrogenase) form xanthine oxidase, which blocks essential defensive mechanisms against oxidative stress.

Lipid peroxidation via myeloperoxidase causes degradation of unsaturated fatty acids and alters the structure of myelin, producing an immunologic response, and demyelination of CNS lipids follows. Toxicity is multi-factorial, resulting from a permutation of tissue hypoxia, direct CO-mediated damage at the cellular level, and consequent harm due to oxidative stress, triggering of inflammatory cascades, and lipid peroxidation. Organs with the highest oxygen demand, the brain and heart, are the most susceptible to the ischaemic injuries. The deleterious effects on the heart, specifically, can vary extensively as the CV health of the exposed person deeply affects redeeming mechanisms. In hypoxaemia, cardiac output increases to maintain oxygen delivery to the brain, as with anaemia or at altitude. With sustained and progressive hypoxaemia, cardiac output will maximize and cannot compensate for the reduced oxygen-carrying capacity in carboxyhaemoglobinemia. Demand ischaemia following decrease of cardiac output results, worsening cardiac ischaemia. This is a brutal cycle, proliferating cerebral and peripheral ischaemia as well. Hence, loss of consciousness, apparently owing to decreased cardiac output and/or cerebral ischaemia, has been recognized as a strong interpreter of severe toxicity. CO exposure has a harmful effect in utero. The foetus is much more sensitive to hypoxia and direct toxic effects at cellular level. Foetal haemoglobin has a higher affinity for oxygen. Carboxyhaemoglobin further over stresses the left shift, reducing the release of oxygen in the tissues producing intense hypoxia. In order to reduce exposure to CO, it is most important that combustion equipment is properly maintained.

Nitrous Oxide Toxicity: Nitrogen is a colourless, tasteless, and odourless gas that comprises up to 78 percent by volume of air. Nitrogen is usually an inert diatomic gas that has no direct physiologic toxicity. Oxides of nitrogen (nitric oxide and nitrogen dioxides) are gases that can be released from nitrous or nitric acid as a result of the reaction between nitric acid and organic materials, burning of nitrocellulose, as a result of ignitions, and as a breakdown of rocket fuel. Nitrogen dioxide and other oxides of nitrogen are found in a variety of occupational settings. A person may also become exposed to nitrogen oxides from electric arc welding, electroplating, and engraving. Nitrogen oxides are found in engine exhaust and are also produced while filling silos with grain having high nitrite content. Nitric oxide reacts with oxygen to form nitrogen dioxide.

Oxides of nitrogen can be produced by ice resurfacing machines during the burning of propane. Its indoor exposure can be an ice-skating rink with poor ventilation. In 1987, 116 people attending an ice hockey game in Minnesota reported various symptoms from cough to haemoptysis because of exposure to nitrogen dioxide. The classic example of nitrogen dioxide toxicity is known as '*silo filler's disease*'. Silo filler's disease occurs when a patient inhales nitrogen dioxide that forms during the decomposition of silage. Workers with occupation that expose them to nitrogen oxides are normally at risk for its toxicity. They may be unaware of on-going exposures. Longer exposures allow a higher concentration of nitrogen oxides to reach the lower airways, resulting in delayed lower respiratory tract injury. *Silo filler's disease* is an occupational disease that occurs due to the inhalation of nitrogen oxides while filling agricultural grain silos with organic matter, usually corn or other grains.

Nitrous oxide is a colourless and odourless gas popularly known as 'laughing gas'. When breathed in, it slows down the body's reaction time, which results in a calm, excited feeling. It is usually used for treating pain and also functions as a mild sedative. It is occasionally used before dental procedures to stimulate relaxation and decrease anxiety. As a sedative, nitrous oxide works fast, but it doesn't take long for the effects to disappear.

Health Implications and Symptoms: Nitrous oxide is safe; but, like any other drug, it may have side effects. Common short-term side effects include:

- Dizziness
- Excessive sweating
- Fatigue
- Nausea
- Shivering
- Vomiting

Some people may experience illusions or sound distortion after breathing this gas. Oxygen is sometimes administered along with nitrous oxide. Regardless of the fact that the gas is safe and used clinically, there's a risk of overdose. This can occur due to long-term exposure and signs of a possible overdose may include:

- Blue fingers, toes, and lips
- Breathlessness, coughing, or difficulty breathing

- Fast heart rate
- Hang-up or illusions
- Irritation of the nose, eyes, and throat
- Obstructing or stiffness in the chest
- Seizures

An increase in blood pressure may also occur, which raises the risk of a stroke or heart attack. A large dose of nitrous oxide without sufficient oxygen may result in brain damage. If left unattended, an overdose can cause coma or death.

Aetiology and Pathophysiology: Nitrogen oxides are irritant gases with low water solubility. Because of low water solubility of nitrogen oxides there are delayed-onset pulmonary effects. Nitrogen dioxide and other oxides of nitrogen damage lung tissue through the ultimate generation of reactive nitrogen-derived free radicals. Moreover, on contact with water, oxides of nitrogen produce nitric acid, resulting in irritation or damage to the lung tissue. Nitrogen oxide is low water-soluble gas and is, therefore, able to penetrate the distal bronchioles and adjacent alveoli. Nitrogen dioxide is believed to cause a direct injury to the alveolar epithelial cells via the generation of toxic free radicals, which may lead to diffuse alveolar injury damage. With increasing concentration exposures, there is an increased risk of pulmonary oedema. Toxic pneumonitis and bronchiolitis can develop at exposure levels of 25 to 100 ppm. Exposures greater than 150 ppm are usually fatal due to bronchiolitis obliterans, chemical pneumonitis, and pulmonary oedema. Nitrogen dioxide toxicity can be described as a triphasic illness. The initial presentation may consist of cough, wheezing, dyspnoea, chest pain, fever, sweating, and weakness. In the second phase, the patient may be comparatively asymptomatic. The third phase develops two to eight weeks later and a patient may develop bronchiolitis obliterans.

Sulphur Dioxide Toxicity: Sulphur dioxide (SO_2) is a colourless gas with a strong, annoying odour. It is produced during the burning of fossil fuels and smelting of mineral ores containing sulphur. Volcanic eruptions can be a significant natural source of SO_2 emissions. When SO_2 combines with water and air, it forms H_2SO_4, which is the main constituent of acid rain. Acid rain can cause deforestation, acidify waterways and damage aquatic life, and corrode building materials and paints.

Health Implications and Symptoms: SO_2 affects the respiratory system, particularly lung function, and can irritate the eyes. SO_2 irritates the respiratory tract and increases the risk of infections. It causes coughing and mucous secretion and intensifies conditions such as asthma and chronic bronchitis. Most of the SO_2 that enters the upper respiratory tract through the nose and mouth is absorbed through the mucous membrane. In the body, it is metabolized in the liver and excreted in the urine. Therefore, very little or almost no SO_2 stores in the body and harm to internal organs is minimal. Besides being absorbed by the respiratory tract, bacteria in the nose and throat produce various substances that bind SO_2 and inactivate it.

The effects of SO_2 can be divided into short-term effects owing to sudden pollution, which continues for a few minutes or hours, and long-term effects occur when the pollution continues for days, months, or even years. The short-term effects at low concentrations are chiefly irritation of the eyes, nose, and throat and probably headaches. At higher levels, coughing may be noticed, mainly in people with lung disease. Symptoms appear the moment the pollution reaches levels that affect the individual, but also disappear once the pollution goes away. The long-term effects of SO_2 cause permanent respiratory symptoms, such as cough, runny nose, and asthma. SO_2 pollution can cause retarded growth of foetuses in pregnant women and also results in premature births.

Ozone Toxicity: Ozone usually occurs in a gaseous state as three atoms of oxygen (O) linked in a cyclic structure and is a by-product of water purification, bleaching, and any process generating a spark or electric arc in the presence of oxygen. Ozone is also found in the atmosphere, with higher altitudes having higher levels of ozone. Ozone is also an environmental air pollutant together with SO_2 and PM. Ozone can react with air and create NO_2, another air pollutant. Despite this, ozone can be produced by medical devices for therapeutic purposes. Ozone has wide applications:

- Regulating post-operative pain after dental extraction
- Mending inner ear damage caused by acoustic trauma
- Decreasing coronary stent restenosis
- Enhancing methicillin-resistant *Staphylococcus aureus* elimination in mediastinitis in combination with antibiotics
- Ozone is used in the pre-treatment of textile wastewater
- Ozone is used in many industries. It is used for purifying air and drinking water, in industrial waste treatment, oils, bleaching and waxes, and to make other chemicals.

The following workers are at risk of being exposed to ozone:

- Outdoor workers in areas with high levels of ozone
- Factory workers in paper and pulp mills
- Workers in wastewater treatment plants
- Fisheries workers involved in treating storage water

Ozone reacts with chemicals to produce other potentially toxic substances such as formaldehyde. Ozone is an important component of smog. It is a highly reactive and unstable gas which can damage living cells. Ozone is formed in the atmosphere through complex reactions between chemicals directly emitted from vehicles, industrial plants, consumer products, and many other sources. Hydrocarbons and nitrogen oxide gases react in the presence of sunlight to form ozone. Hot, sunshiny, and calm weather stimulates formation of ozone. Ozone has a pungent odour, like chlorine bleach, and it can be detected after lightning strikes or during electrical discharges. Ozone as an air pollutant is produced close to the ground level, where people live, and breathe. A layer of ozone high up in the atmosphere is called stratospheric ozone, which prevents the entry of ultraviolet light to the Earth's atmosphere. Without stratospheric ozone, plant and animal life would be seriously harmed. Ozone reacts with surfaces as it enters the indoor environment, usually resulting in lower levels indoors than outdoors. Equipment such as photocopiers, laser printers, and some air purifiers can emit ozone indoors as well. Once inside, depending on its concentration ozone can cause harmful health effects and damage materials.

Ozone can damage the respiratory tract tissues, causing inflammation and irritation, and results in symptoms such as coughing, chest tightness, and worsening of asthma symptoms. Exposure to ozone can reduce the volume of air that the lungs breathe in and cause shortness of breath. Children, youngsters, and adults, who exercise or work outdoors, where ozone concentration is high, are at a higher risk of this pollutant. Ozone exposure reduces the productivity of plants, damaging cells and causing destruction of leaf tissue. Consequently, ozone exposure decreases the plants' ability to photosynthesize. This weakens plants, making them vulnerable to disease, pests, cold and drought. Ozone also decreases crop and timber yields. Moreover, ozone disturbs the stability of ecosystems. Besides, ozone exposure decreases the production of roots, seeds, fruit, and other plant constituents. Ozone causes considerable damage to various materials such as rubber, plastics, fabrics, paint, and metals. Exposure to ozone gradually damages both the functional and aesthetic qualities of materials and products, and reduces their life spans.

Aetiology and Pathophysiology: Exposure to ozone is probably unintended owing to environmental sources both indoor and outdoor. Despite its decreased presence, ozone can react with many indoor chemicals such as those used for wood flooring, carpeting, and perfume and create potentially harmful compounds. Route of exposure governs the toxic effect of ozone as the skin is somewhat tolerant, while the respiratory system is intolerant and can show harmful effects even at low ambient environmental concentrations. Toxic effects occur through free radicals and oxidation, or through radical-dependent pathways. Besides generation of free radicals, ozone can deplete antioxidants. Exposure to ozone may cause headaches, coughing, dry throat, shortness of breath, heaviness in chest, and fluid in the lungs. Higher exposure can lead to more severe symptoms. Chronic exposure causes asthma, while recurrent exposure causes permanent scar in lung tissue.

Cyanide Toxicity: Cyanides are fast-acting lethal poisons. Cyanides were used as chemical weapons for the first time in the First World War. Lower levels of cyanides are found in nature and in products commonly consumed or used. Some bacteria, fungi, and algae can produce cyanides. Cyanides are also found in cigarette smoke, vehicle exhaust, and in eatables for instance spinach, bamboo shoots, almonds, lima beans, fruit pits, and tapioca. Cyanide and cyanide-containing compounds are used in pesticides and fumigants, plastics, electroplating, photo developing, and mining. Dye and pharmaceutical companies also use cyanides.

Industrial processes, such as iron and steel production, wastewater treatment produce cyanides. Cyanogen chloride is produced during water chlorination.

People may be exposed to low levels of cyanides in their daily lives from foods, smoking, and other sources. Eating or drinking cyanide-containing foods has health implications. Inhaling cyanide gas, mainly in a badly aerated space, has the highest possible harm. Deadly exposures to cyanides result from accidents or deliberate actions. Owing to their quick-acting property, cyanides may be used in terrorism.

There are many chemical forms of cyanide. Hydrogen cyanide is a pale blue or colourless liquid at room temperature and is a colourless gas at higher temperature. It has a bitter almond odour. Sodium cyanide and potassium cyanide are white powders which may have a bitter almond-like odour. Chemicals like cyanogens can generate cyanides. Cyanogen chloride is a colourless liquefied gas that is heavier than air and has a strong odour.

After exposure, cyanide rapidly goes into the bloodstream. The body handles small amounts of cyanide in a different way than large amounts. In small dosage, cyanide in the body can be changed into thiocyanate, which is less detrimental and is expelled in urine. Cyanide in small amounts can also combine with another chemical to form vitamin B12, which helps maintain healthy nerve and red blood cells. The body's ability to change cyanide into thiocyanate is exhausted in large doses. A large dose of cyanide prevents cells from using oxygen and ultimately the cells die. The heart, respiratory system, and central nervous system are most vulnerable to cyanide poisoning. The health implications of cyanide exposure can begin in seconds. Some signs and symptoms of such exposures are:

- Cardiac arrest
- Gasping for air and difficulty breathing
- Headache
- Loss of consciousness
- Nausea
- Seizures
- Weakness and confusion

The severity of health consequences depends upon the route and duration of exposure, dose, and type/ variety of cyanide. Acute cyanide poisoning is relatively rare, but has instantaneous, often serious effects. It may result in difficulty breathing, seizure, loss of consciousness, and cardiac arrest. In chronic cyanide poisoning, symptoms are often gradual and increase in severity with the passage of time. Early symptoms may include:

- Bright red flush
- Drowsiness
- Headache
- Nausea
- Vertigo
- Vomiting

Additional symptoms may include:

- Clammy skin
- Convulsions
- Dilated pupils
- Slower, shallower breaths
- Weaker, more rapid pulse

If the person remains undiagnosed and unattended, it can lead to:

- Blue lips, face, and extremities
- Decreased body temperature
- Slow, irregular heart rate
- Coma
- Death

Aetiology and Pathophysiology: Intravenous and breathing in cyanide produce a faster onset of signs and symptoms than exposure via oral or transdermal route. The toxicity of cyanide is associated mostly to the termination of aerobic cell metabolism. Cyanide reversibly binds to the ferric ions cytochrome oxidase in mitochondria. This efficiently stops cellular respiration by obstructing the reduction of oxygen to water. The main effect of cyanide is that it obstructs oxidative phosphorylation, a process where oxygen is utilized for the production of essential cellular energy in form of ATP. It does so by binding to the enzyme cytochrome c oxidase and blocking the mitochondrial transport chain. Afterward, cellular hypoxia and depletion of ATP occur, leading to metabolic acidosis. The use of oxygen by the tissue occurs and is followed by the diminishing of vital functions. Cyanide rapidly gets absorbed through the respiratory tract and mucous membranes as well as the gastrointestinal tract and skin. Signs and symptoms start when the blood cyanide concentration is approximately 40 mol/L.

Thus, implications of air pollutants on living organisms are not only limited to human and animal health but the environment as a whole. Diverse topographical conditions, global climate conditions, and ecological disparities affect human health and the environment including the biodiversity. Ecologically, air pollution can cause severe environmental damage to groundwater, soil, and air. Studies on the connection between air pollution and reducing species diversity reveal the harmful effects of environmental pollutants on the extinction of animals and plant species. Air suspended toxicants have reproductive implications in animals. Acid rain, temperature upturn, and global climate changes owing to the emissions of greenhouse gases in the atmosphere are other main ecological impacts of air pollution.

Every material in the air that could affect human health or have an intense impact on the environment is defined as an air pollutant. According to the WHO, particle pollution, ground-level O_3, CO, sulphur oxides, nitrogen oxides, and lead (Pb) are the six major air pollutants which harm human health and the ecosystem. Particle pollutants form a major share of air pollutants. They are basically a combination of particles found in the air. Particle pollution is linked with most pulmonary and cardiac-associated morbidity and mortality.

The size of particle pollutants is directly linked with the beginning and progression of lung and heart diseases. Particles of smaller size reach the lower respiratory tract and have greater potential for causing lung and heart diseases. Depending on the level of exposure, particulate pollutants may cause mild to severe illnesses. Long-term exposure to ambient PM concentrations leads to reduced life expectancy. The increase of cardiopulmonary and lung cancer mortality is the main reason for reduced life expectancy. Reduced lung functions in children and adults leading to asthmatic bronchitis and chronic obstructive pulmonary disease (COPD) are serious health implications which prompt reduced life expectancy.

Transmission of airborne diseases can be greatly reduced by practicing social and respiratory protocol. Staying home during illness, minimizing contact with an ill person, and wearing a mask, can greatly reduce the transmission. Hand washing can decrease spreading of germ-containing droplets that come in contact with hands from surfaces contaminated with secretions. Environmental controls and engineering substitutes help decrease transmission of water droplet aerosolized pathogens.

BIBLIOGRAPHY

Ashurst, J. and Wasson, M. (2011) Methemoglobinemia: A systematic review of the pathophysiology, detection, and treatment. *Delaware Medical Journal* 83(7):203–208.

Benner, J. P., Lawrence D. and Brady, W. (2009) Smoke signals: Recognition and treatment of combustion-induced cyanide toxicity. *Journal of Electronic Materials* 34(10):56–63.

Brooks, S. M. (2013) Upper and lower airways obstruction following an inhalation injury. *Journal of Occupational and Environmental Medicine* 55(5):594–596.

Buckey, J. C. (2019) Use of gases to treat cochlear conditions. *Frontier in Cellular Neuroscience* 13:155.

Elvis, A. M. and Ekta, J. S. (2011) Ozone therapy: A clinical review. *Journal of Natural Science, Biology and Medicine* 2(1):66–70.

Ernst, A. and Zibrak, J. D. (1998) Carbon monoxide poisoning. *New England Journal of Medicine* 339(22):1603–1608.

Goodman, J. E., *et al.* (2018) Short-term ozone exposure and asthma severity: Weight-of-evidence analysis. *Environmental Research* 160:391–397.

Gorguner, M. and Akgun, M. (2010) Acute inhalation injury. *Eurasian Journal of Medicine* 42(1):28–35.

Hampson, N. B. and Weaver, L. K. (2007) Carbon monoxide poisoning: A new incidence for an old disease. *Undersea and Hyperbaric Medicine* 34(3):163–168.

Henry, C. R., *et al.* (2006) Myocardial injury and long-term mortality following moderate to severe carbon monoxide poisoning. *Journal of American Medical Association* 295(4): 398–402.

Hernberg, S. (1992) *Introduction to Occupational Epidemiology*. Philadelphia: Lewis Publishers.

Holkar, C. R., *et al.* (2016) A critical review on textile wastewater treatments: Possible approaches. *Journal of Environmental Management* 182:351–366.

Huzar, T. F., George, T. and Cross, J. M. (2013) Carbon monoxide and cyanide toxicity: Etiology, pathophysiology and treatment in inhalation injury. *Expert Review of Respiratory Medicine* 7(2):159–170.

Jayalakshmi, T. K., *et al.* (2009) Acute lung injury following exposure to nitric acid. *Lung India* 26(4):149–151.

Jung, S. J., Mehta, J. S. and Tong, L. (2018) Effects of environment pollution on the ocular surface. *Ocular Surface* 16(2): 198–205.

Kelly, F. J. and Mudway, I. S. (2003) Protein oxidation at the air-lung interface. *Amino Acids* 25(3–4):375–396.

Kinoshita, H., *et al.* (2020) Carbon monoxide poisoning. *Toxicology Reports* 7:169–173.

Levy, B. S. and Wegman, D. H. (1994) *Occupational Health: Recognizing and Preventing Work-Related Disease*. Boston: Little Brown.

Li, X., *et al.* (2019) Effects of ambient ozone concentrations with different averaging times on asthma exacerbations: A meta-analysis. *Science of Total Environment* 691:549–561.

Lindsley, W. G., *et al.* (2014) Efficacy of face shields against cough aerosol droplets from a cough simulator. *Journal of Occupational and Environmental Hygiene* 11(8):509–518.

McKay, C. A. (2014) Toxin-induced respiratory distress. *Emergency Medicine Clinics of North America* 32(1):127–147.

Meaden, C. W., Kashani, J. S. and Vetrano, S. (2019) Pulmonary edema occurring after nitric acid exposure. *Case Reports in Emergency Medicine*.

O'Brien, D. J., Walsh, D. W., Terriff, C. M. and Hall, A. H. (2011) Empiric management of cyanide toxicity associated with smoke inhalation. *Prehospital and Disaster Medicine* 26(5):374–382.

Oktem, Y. A., *et al.* (2019) Chloride or sulfate? Consequences for ozonation of textile wastewater. *Journal of Environmental Management* 247:749–755.

Pauluhn, J. (2016) Risk assessment in combustion toxicology: Should carbon dioxide be recognized as a modifier of toxicity or separate toxicological entity? *Toxicology Letters* 16(262):142–152.

Prockop, L. D. and Chichkova, R. I. (2007) Carbon monoxide intoxication: an updated review. *Journal of Neuroscience* 262(1–2):122–130.

Rosenstock, L. and Cullen, M. R. (1994) *Textbook of Clinical Occupational and Environmental Medicine*. Philadelphia: Saunders.

Rowland, F. S. (2006) Stratospheric ozone depletion. *Philosophical Transactions of the Royal Society B: Biological Sciences* 361(1469):769–790.

Ruth-Sahd, L. A. and White, K. A. (2009) Bronchiolitis obliterans organizing pneumonia. *Dimension of Critical Care Nursing* 28(5):204–208.

Skold, A., Cosco, D. L. and Klein, R. (2011) Methemoglobinemia: pathogenesis, diagnosis, and management. *South Medical Journal* 104(11):757–761.

Tang, J. W., *et al.* (2006) Factors involved in the aerosol transmission of infection and control of ventilation in healthcare premises. *Journal of Hospital Infection* 64(2):100–114.

Torne, R., Soyer, H. P., Leb, G. and Kerl, H. (1991) Skin lesions in carbon monoxide intoxication. *Dermatologica* 183(3):212–215.

Weschler, C. J. (2006) Ozone's impact on public health: contributions from indoor exposures to ozone and products of ozone-initiated chemistry. *Environmental Health Perspectives* 114(10):1489–1496.

11 Natural Disasters and Health

"We learn from every natural disaster. Whether it's a fire or a flood, we learn something from it so we can respond to the next one better."

—Malcolm Turnbull

FACT FILE

- "Earthquakes" are disasters that cause destruction of man-made structures and instigate other natural disasters such as tsunamis, avalanches, and landslides
- Landslides often accompany earthquakes, floods, storm surges, hurricanes, wildfires, or volcanic activity
- The penalties to the economy, as well as public health and safety, due to natural hazards, such as droughts, earthquakes, wildfires, hurricanes, volcanic eruptions, and tornadoes, can be devastating
- People who live in low-lying coastal areas are exposed to extreme sea-level events including tsunamis
- The number of deaths due to natural disasters varies from year to year
- Approximately 45,000 people globally died from natural disasters each year over the past decade
- Worldwide, over the past decade, natural disasters accounted for an average of 0.1 percent of total deaths
- During the 20th century there was a significant decline in global deaths from natural disasters. In the early 1900s, the annual average was often in the range of 400,000 to 500,000 deaths
- Worldwide, disasters were responsible for 0.1 percent of deaths over the past decade
- Deaths from natural disasters have seen a large decline over the past century
- Factually, droughts and floods were the most deadly disaster events. Deaths from these events are now very low – the most fatal events today tend to be earthquakes
- Disasters affect those in poverty most seriously: high death tolls tend to be focused in low-to-middle-income nations lacking proper infrastructure to safeguard and respond to events

11.1 INTRODUCTION

Health is one of the key goals and an important benchmark of realization of effective disaster management. Healthcare is a vital factor for survival in the initial

DOI: 10.1201/9781003464785-11

stages of a disaster. When it comes to disaster mitigation, preparedness, and response, hospitals and healthcare professionals need special consideration owing to the vital functions they execute, their high level of occupancy, and the role they play during a disaster. The impacts of disasters could be:

- Direct on the health sector infrastructure, viz. damage to the hospital building
- Loss of or injury to the health personnel
- Destruction or damage to the other infrastructure
- Pressure on the existing resource
- Larger influx of patients

During all phases of a disaster, a systematic approach is desirable to design, implement, monitor, and evaluate these inclusive services. This chapter is focused on the health implications of disasters.

11.2 GENERAL EFFECTS OF DISASTERS ON HEALTH

The term '*disaster*' refers to the natural event that has damaging effects, viz., the loss of life or destruction of buildings.

'*Hazard*' refers to the natural event

'*Vulnerability*' is the susceptibility of a population or system (e.g. a hospital, water supply, and sewage system, or aspects of infrastructure) to the effects of the hazard.

'*Risk*' is the probability that a particular system or population will be affected by hazards is known as the

Hence, risk is a function of the vulnerability and the hazard, and is expressed as follows:

$$\text{Risk} = \text{Vulnerability X Hazard}$$

Though all disasters are unique in that they affect areas with different levels of vulnerability and with distinct social, health, and economic conditions, there are still similarities between disasters. If recognized, these common factors can be used to improve the management of health humanitarian assistance and use of resources (Table 11.1).

It is important to note that:

- civil wars and conflicts produce a distinct set of public health problems and operational restraints
- actual and potential health risks after a disaster don't occur at the same time, rather they arise at different times and differ in significance in a disaster-affected area
- the effects have probable, rather than inevitable, threats to health; for example, the movement of population and other environmental changes

TABLE 11.1
Level of Effects Produced by Natural Disasters

Effect	Earthquake	High Winds (without Flooding)	Tidal Waves/Flash Floods	Slow-onset Floods	Landslides	Volcanoes/Lahars
Damage to healthcare facilities	Severe (structure and equipment)	Severe	Severe but localized	Severe (equipment)	Severe but localized	Severe (structure and equipment)
Damage to water systems	Severe	Light	Severe	Light	Severe but localized	Severe
Death	Many	Few	Many	Few	Many	Many
Food shortage	Rare		Common	Common	Rare	Rare
Increased risk of communicable diseases	Potential risk after major disasters probably due to overcrowding and deteriorating sanitation					
Major population movement	Rare (may occur in heavily damaged urban areas)			Common (usually rare)		
Severe injuries that require extensive treatment	Many	Moderate	Few	Few	Few	Few

increase the risk of disease transmission, although epidemics usually do not result from natural disasters
- there is a relationship between the type of disaster and its impact on health; for instance, earthquakes cause injuries requiring medical care, while floods and tidal waves cause relatively few
- the needs for food, shelter, and primary healthcare are usually not complete because even displaced people often recover some basic needs of life

11.2.1 Health Problems Common to All Natural Disasters

Social Response: After a major natural disaster, behaviour influences generalized panic or stunned waiting. Earthquake survivors often search for rescue activities after an impact and within hours organize themselves into groups to transport the incapacitated to medical posts. Anti-social behaviour such as extensive looting occurs in exceptional circumstances. During warning periods, or after the occurrence of natural disasters, people are reluctant to evacuate, even if their homes are likely to be or have been destroyed (Table 11.2).

Communicable Diseases: Usually natural disasters do not result in a large outbreak of infectious disease, though in certain circumstances they do increase the likelihood of disease transmission. The most commonly observed increase in incidence of disease is due to faecal contamination of water and food; hence, such diseases are mostly enteric.

TABLE 11.2
Disaster-Related Psychological and Physical Response

Emotional Response	Cognitive Response	Physical Response	Interpersonal Response
• Anger • Annoyance • Emotional shock • Fear • Feeling dejected or depressed • Feeling miserable or impossible • Feeling speechless • Guiltiness • Misery • Susceptibility	• Misunderstanding • Difficulty in decision-making • Memory loss • Enquiring spiritual beliefs • Recurrent hallucinations • Self-blame • Trouble in focusing or memorizing things	• Anxiety • Body aches and pains • Fast heartbeat • Headaches • High BP • Increase or decrease in appetite • Insomnia • Lethargy • Rapid shock response • Strain • Vomiting	• Being judgmental • Crying • Feeling suspicious • Feeling rejected and reckless • Increased family clashes • Irritability • Insomnia • Social withdrawal

The threat of outbreak of epidemic is related to population density and displacement. These situations:

- increase the pressure on water and food supplies and the risk of contamination
- disrupt the pre-existing sanitation services, for instance, piped water and sewage, and failure to maintain or restore normal public health programs in the post-disaster period
- increase the vector-borne diseases in some areas due to disturbance of vector control efforts, mainly after heavy rains and floods
- wash away residual insecticides from the buildings and the number of mosquito breeding sites may increase
- brings additional risk of zoonotic infections due to displacement of wild or domesticated animals near human settlements
- in complex disasters where malnourishment, congestion, and scarcity of basic hygiene are common, catastrophic outbreaks of gastroenteritis, triggered by cholera or other diseases occur

Population Displacements: A critical need to provide humanitarian assistance is produced when large, unplanned, or planned population migrations occur. If the inhabitation has been damaged, there may be large population movements as people seek shelter with relatives and friends.

Climatic Exposure: The health hazards of exposure to the elements are not great, even after disasters in temperate climates. As long as the population is dry, reasonably well clothed, and able to find windbreaks, death from exposure does not appear to be a major risk in Latin America and the Caribbean. The need to provide emergency shelter therefore varies greatly with local conditions.

Food and Nutrition: Food scarcity is the instantaneous outcome of disaster that may arise in two ways. Damage of food stock in the disaster area may affect the availability of food, or disrupt the public distribution systems limiting access to food, even if there is no actual dearth. Widespread food scarcities are sufficient to cause nutritional deficiency problems after natural disasters. Flooding and sea surges often damage household food stocks and crops, disrupt distribution, and cause major scarcities. In prolonged droughts, the destitute, and migrants may be totally dependent on outside food sources for indefinite time period. Based on the nutritional status of population, particularly of more susceptible groups such as pregnant or lactating women, children, and the elderly, it may be essential to introduce emergency feeding programs.

Water Supply and Sanitation: Drinking water supply and sewage systems are mostly vulnerable to natural hazards and the disturbances that occur pose serious health risks. The systems are exposed to a variety of hazards. Deterioration of drinkable water and problems in the disposal of excreta and other wastes worsens sanitation, furthering favourable conditions for spreading of enteric and other diseases, immediately following disasters, viz.:

- Acute public health problems
- Depression
- Mental health anxiety
- Neuroses

Waning Healthcare Infrastructure: Natural disasters cause serious damage to healthcare amenities including water supply and sewage systems, which has a direct impact on the health of the population dependent on these services. In case of physically unsafe hospitals and healthcare centres, natural disasters threaten the life of occupants of buildings and limit the capacity to provide health services to disaster victims.

11.2.2 Direct Effects of Natural Disasters

Natural disasters are complex happenings in which people are exposed to a variety of risks and hazards. Every disaster situation is exclusive in its own way and reveals intermittent challenges to sufferers and rescue emergency personnel alike. On the one hand, each disaster must be assessed independently to identify the special features of the situation at hand. In this manner, one avoids the common mistake of preparing for the last disaster situation as opposed to anticipating the next one. On the other hand, certain disaster situations do follow general patterns and develop along similar paths. It is vital to appreciate these subtle patterns in order to provide community planners and allied health professionals with a foundation to design a comprehensive emergency response plan.

A fine balance must be maintained between learning from the mistakes and lessons of the past, and resisting the temptation of simply approaching a situation 'the way it has always been done'. Generally speaking, certain disasters lead to certain types of injuries more than others. This can be an important fact to bear in mind when planning an emergency response, taking stock of available medical supplies, or estimating the needs of a community or geographical area. It is crucial, however, to be conscious that injury types are not exclusive to any one situation. Indeed the sheer scale and complexity of a natural disaster may lead to many smaller disaster situations; each one with its own individual characteristics and challenges.

An example of a large-scale catastrophe causing many smaller emergency situations is a large-scale flood which in turn causes a chemical spill from a water-logged factory, a landslide burying several homes, drinking water reservoir contamination, and the collapse of a downtown building. As a basis for planning, it is nevertheless useful to consider the types of injuries the majority of the victims will incur in order to evaluate the immediate needs of the disaster response team. Droughts The immediate emergency effects of a drought are subtle when compared to those brought on by natural disasters such as tornadoes or hurricanes. In a region that has been severely affected by drought, mortality may increase sharply due to protein malnutrition (kwashiorkor) or calorie malnutrition (marasmus). Certain vitamin deficiencies, such as a lack of Vitamin A, can lead to specific consequences such as xerophthalmia and child blindness. Long-standing malnutrition can easily lead to increased rates of disease and mortality, and limit the general population's functionality.

In some cases, mass movements of people spurred by long-standing drought and food shortages can lead to over-crowding and collectively poor hygiene. Over-crowding can easily lead to an increase in the transmission rates of communicable diseases such as tuberculosis or gastro-intestinal infections.

Earthquakes: Risk of injury in open areas or in the countryside is much lower as compared to thickly populated areas. Furthermore, severity of injury is inversely related to the distance from the epicentre of the earthquake. Earthquakes induce:

- high level of mortality due to crush injuries from falling objects both indoors or in close proximity to structures
- greater incidence of trauma to the pelvis, thorax, and spine in case of night earthquake
- severe damage to internal organs coinciding with severe internal bleeding
- injuries and deaths are generally increased with the magnitude of the earthquake, increased ground motion, and structural damage
- daytime earthquake causes injuries of the extremities with comorbid lacerations, severe external bleeding, and crush injuries including compartment syndrome
- amputations, vascular stabilization, orthopaedic stabilization, and debridement and/or dressing of severe open wounds
- patients suffering from crush injuries are at high risk of developing hypovolemic shock, hyperkalemia, and renal failure, and have a greater chance of having a fatal cardiac arrhythmia or myocardial infarction

Fires: Fire is another major concern after the disaster. On the basis of size and magnitude of fires, burn injuries, and respiratory problems due to inhalation of smoke is a major concern. The highest health impact of a forest fire is its effect on the surrounding air quality. Because of appropriate local conditions, many smaller fires can add to poor air quality of a particular area. Fire causes respiratory problems or worsens existing conditions. Burn injuries from forest fires are associated with forest firefighting crews. Depending on the wind conditions, forest fires spread fast and change direction quickly which can entrap the firefighters and private citizens. During the large forest fire, animal attacks and/or bites also increase. Depending on the proximity of a forest fire to a population, many wild animals take flight and come in contact with human beings. Injuries in a large-scale fire are burn injuries and deaths linked with asphyxiation. Common problems of burn injuries include hypovolemic shock, massive infection, and sepsis.

Floods: Drowning is probably the greatest risk of mortality from a flood. In many nations, floods account for more annual deaths than other natural disasters. The highest number of deaths and injuries occur mainly when there is no cautioning of a forthcoming flood. This can occur in the case of flash flooding, the collapse of a dam, or from the action of a tidal wave due to a distant or even sub-oceanic earthquake.

Consistently, individuals underestimate the power of moving water leading to what could have been many preventable deaths and injuries. In the best of times, it is difficult to estimate the average depth of opaque and fast-moving water; and it can be next to impossible at dusk or in the middle of the night. It takes less than two feet of moving water to float a large vehicle such as a school bus, and only between three and six inches of fast-moving water to sweep a large man off of his feet. Second only to drowning, exposure to the elements accounts for a large percentage of the deaths and critical injuries that occur in floods. In many cases, individuals who are caught in rising floodwaters wait for rescue in any refuge that can be found including trees, tops of buildings, and automobiles. Depending on the extent of the flooding and the availability of rescue personnel, people may spend hours to days openly exposed to inclement weather. The lower the ambient temperature falls below 15°C, the greater the risk of accidental hypothermia. Blunt trauma injuries are not uncommon in floods due to the amount of debris that may be caught in the moving floodwaters along with the unsuspecting victims. Injuries in this case resemble projectile injuries and commonly include extremity and torso fractures, lacerations, and severe bruising.

Heat Waves: Heat waves are known as the silent natural disaster. The immediate health effects of a heat wave are perceptible among vulnerable populations including the elderly, young, and sick and all are vulnerable to heat stress, which can ultimately take a patient from heat exhaustion to a fatal heat stroke. However, it is important to note that the young and healthy are also vulnerable to heat illness if the proper precautions are not taken. Heat illnesses are preventable by remaining in hot weather conditions for a short duration. Maintaining fluid balance by consuming plenty of liquids and restricting alcoholic or caffeinated beverages prevents illnesses caused by excessive heat. Treatment of advanced stages of heat illness, such as heat stroke, includes rapid cooling of the body together with fluid and electrolyte replacement. The body temperature must be checked to protect against hyperthermia or inadvertent hypothermia. The mortality rate for heat stroke is linked with the duration and severity of hyperthermia and suitability of diagnosis and treatment.

Cyclones, Hurricanes, and Typhoons: In the last few decades, constant population growth together with development of susceptible coastal areas has increased hurricane-related deaths, injuries, and economic penalties. In a hurricane, the highest mortality arises from the secondary disasters such as small tornadoes, flash flooding, and storm surges that have been prompted. In coastal regions, the level of a hurricane's storm surge is one of the strongest predictors of mortality. Wind is the second deadliest aspect of a hurricane, which often causes property damage resulting in collapse of houses and other wooden structures. Rupturing of windows or doors due to flying objects or wind pressure are common damaging signs. Crush injuries are also common in severe storms. The most common non-fatal traumatic injury in a hurricane is superficial tears due to hovering glass and other debris.

Tornadoes: The foremost cause of death and permanent injury in a tornado is cranio-cerebral injury due to projectiles hastened by tornado winds. Crush injuries due to disintegrating buildings or very large airborne debris are also frequent.

Common non-fatal injuries include fractures, penetrating trauma, tears, and other soft tissue injuries. Cuts, bruises, scrapes, perforations, and musculoskeletal strain account for over half of the total injuries. Most fatalities suffer due to multiple wounds and many soft tissue injuries occur in exposed skin, for example, the head and neck. Tornado victims also show a characteristic abrasion pattern on exposed skin that is fine particles of soil, mud, sand, and water which strike the body at high speed. Wound contamination, and succeeding infection, seems to be a major cause of post-operative sepsis, which is a multiple organ dysfunction syndrome that leads to multiple system failure.

Volcanoes: Volcanic eruptions have instant life-threatening health effects as they emit tonnes of airborne pollutants in the atmosphere. Like smoke from large forest fires, the airborne pollutants cause respiratory diseases or deteriorate the existing situation. After volcanic eruption, the atmosphere is filled with tonnes of ash and poisonous gases. Toxic volcanic gases such as CO_2, CO, and H_2SO_4 cause acute respiratory distress syndrome, pulmonary oedema, irritant conjunctivitis, joint pain, and muscle weakness. Blisters due to superheated steam from secondary fires initiated by the eruptions are also common. In many instances landslides occur together with volcanic eruptions. Mudslides, which are normally seen in overflowing states, can crush injuries, causing severe internal bleeding, multiple organ dysfunction syndrome, and asphyxia.

Winter Storms: The instant effect of a severe winter storm is generally felt in interruption of traffic patterns and increasing automobile mishaps and traffic collisions, which can cause:

- Bruising
- Fractures
- Head injuries
- Life-threatening bruising of thorax and abdomen
- Orthopaedic injury
- Trauma
- Vascular compromise

Individuals may suffer due to frostbite after prolonged exposure to unusual cold climatic conditions. Severe cases may require amputation. As power lines and communication systems are generally interrupted due to severe winter storm, death from CO poisoning and hypothermia is of a great concern. Moreover, death and injury from fires are more common in winter storms as people leave candles, fireplaces, and heaters burning throughout the night. Also, when sedentary individuals venture out into winter storm to affect repairs or clear snow from roofs, the incidence of angina and acute myocardial infarctions increases intensely.

11.2.3 Indirect Effects of Natural Disasters

Besides the immediate trauma and injuries felt by the victims of natural disasters, studies have revealed numerous secondary medical conditions with a higher incidence in the critical hours and days of recovery period. In many cases, the secondary medical conditions are attributed to the stress. Disaster stress varies from situation to situation and each individual is vulnerable to different types and levels. Table 11.3 shows the age-wise psychological and physical response in the post-disaster phase.

TABLE 11.3
Age-wise Psychological and Physical Response in the Post-disaster Phase

Response among Children	Response among Adolescents	Response among Adults	Response among Elderly People
• Violent behaviour at home or school • Baby talk • Become submissive and silent • Clinging to parent • Competition with younger siblings for parental attention • Fear of darkness • Anxious about weather, security, relapse • Horrified of new circumstances • Annoyances or other grievances • Irritability • Loss of bladder or bowel control, constipation • Loss of attention; poor concentration in school • Increased or decreased appetite • Night terrors, hallucinations, fear of darkness • Escaping school • Separation anxiety • Stammering • Contemplates frightening moments • Thumb-sucking • Withdrawal from peers	• Anxiety • Attention-seeking behaviours • Avoidant behaviour • Bowel problems • Changes in appetite • Changes in peer group or friends • Decreased energy level • Fighting • Headaches • Insomnia • Irresponsible and/ or delinquent behaviour • Loss of interest • Loss of interest in social activities • Pains • Personal isolation • Poor performance • Psychosomatic complaints • Skin eruptions • Use of alcohol and drugs • Withdrawal	• Annoyance • Anxiety • Avoidance of reminders • Changes in appetite • Crying easily • Depression • Deteriorating chronic conditions • Excessive activity level • Exhaustion • Fatigue • Gastrointestinal distress • Grief • Guilt • Hyper-vigilance • Increased conflicts with family • Ineptness • Irritability • Isolation • Misery • Mood swings • Self-doubt • Sleep problems • Somatic complaints • Withdrawal	• Anxiety • Apathy • Apathy • Appetite and sleep problems • Bad temper • Decline in physical health • Depression • Depression about fatalities • Deterioration of chronic infections • Displeasure • Distrust • Irritation • Memory loss • Misunderstanding • Need of Multiple-medication • Perplexity • Physical complaints • Somatic symptoms • Unwillingness to leave home • Withdrawal

Usually mass evacuation of communities leads to total disruption of an individual's personal coping mechanisms. People find themselves thrown from their homes, perhaps quartering in temporary shelters. As temporary shelters are places of last resort, people remain vulnerable to the lack of information and control given them. Along with heart attacks, other cardiovascular complications are gradually seen after natural disasters such as unstable angina and fatal arrhythmias. In many instances, the effect of increased stress load is compounded with the disruption of regular medical services for pre-existing comorbidities.

In some cases, respiratory disorders such as allergies and asthma worsen after a natural disaster. This is mainly true if there has been large-scale release of pollutants into the atmosphere. Interestingly, this seems to be more detrimental to individuals with pre-existing asthmatic or bronchial conditions including rescue and recovery workers. Respiratory infections show a considerable increase in days to weeks after a disaster. This apparent shift in illness is ascribed to the transmission of infectious diseases. While the stress of a natural disaster is felt instantly, the impacts on the health take days to weeks to appear. Many patients suffer from psychological disorders such as post-traumatic stress disorder (PTSD) or general anxiety disorder (GAD) after a disaster event. In many instances victims and survivors suffer due to symptoms, like night terrors, sudden fears, grief, misery, guilt, sleeplessness, loss of appetite, or hallucinations. Psychological rescue from lapses in mental health, brought on by disastrous situations depends on timely recognition of faint symptoms and accessibility of the suitable resources which can promote healing.

BIBLIOGRAPHY

(1977) *Manual for Disaster Relief Work*. New York: Churchill, Livingstone.

(1989) Coping with Natural Disasters: The Role of Local Health Personnel and the Community. Geneva: World Health Organization.

(1999) Rapid Health Assessment Protocols for Emergencies. Geneva: World Health Organisation.

(2000) Natural Disasters – Protecting the Public Health. Pan American Health Organization.

Bayley, J. (1991) Health and safety at work. *British Dental Journal* 170(10):364–365.

Bohonos, J. J. and Hogan, D. E. (1999) The medical impact of tornadoes in North America. *The Journal of Emergency Medicine* 19(1):67–73.

Cutler, R. (1991) Health and safety at work. *British Dental Journal* 170(7): 51.

Dotto, L. (2000) *Storm Warning – Gambling With the Climate of Our Planet Disease and Death: Human Health and Climate Change*. Doubleday Canada Limited.

Greenoough, G. *et al.* (2001) The potential impacts of climate variability and change on health impacts on extreme weather events in the United States. *Environmental Health Perspectives* 109(2):191–198.

Hernberg, S. (1992) *Introduction to Occupational Epidemiology*. Philadelphia: Lewis Publishers.

Iwan, W. D. and Cluff, L. S. *et al.* (1999) Mitigation emerges as major strategy for reducing losses caused by Natural Disasters. *Science* 284(2422):1943–1947.

Levy, B. S. and Wegman, D. H. (1994) *Occupational Health: Recognizing and Preventing Work-Related Disease*. Boston: Little Brown.

Nichols, T. (1998) Health and safety at work. *Work, Employment & Society* 12(2):367–374.

Peek-Asa, C. *et al.* (2000) GIS mapping of earthquake-related deaths and hospital admissions from the 1994 Northridge, California, Earthquake. *Annals of Epidemiology* 10(1):5–13.
Rosenstock, L. and Cullen, M. R. (1994) *Textbook of Clinical Occupational and Environmental Medicine*. Philadelphia: Saunders.
Scott, R. M. (2020) *Chemical Hazards in the Workplace* (e-book). CRC Press.
Spurlock, B. (2017) *Physical Hazards of the Workplace*. CRC Press.
Wijkman, A. and Timberlake, L. (1984) *Natural Disasters: Acts of God or Acts of Man.* London, Washington, DC: International Institute for Environment and Development.
Wilson, H. G. E. and Agius, R. M. (1994) Health and safety at work. *BMJ* 309(6948):198–199.

Index